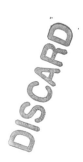

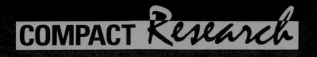

COMPACT *Research*

Sleep Disorders

Hal Marcovitz

Diseases and Disorders

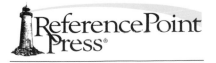

ReferencePoint
Press®

San Diego, CA

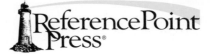

For more information, contact:
ReferencePoint Press, Inc.
PO Box 27779
San Diego, CA 92198
www. ReferencePointPress.com

Picture credits:
Maury Aaseng: 33–36, 49–51, 64–67, 82–83
AP Images: 11, 14

LIBRARY OF CONGRESS CATALOGING-IN-PUBLICATION DATA

Marcovitz, Hal.
  Sleep disorders / by Hal Marcovitz.
    p. cm. — (Compact research series)
  Includes bibliographical references and index.
  ISBN-13: 978-1-60152-071-5 (hardback)
  ISBN-10: 1-60152-071-9 (hardback)
  1. Sleep disorders—Popular works. I. Title.
  RC547.M367 2008
  616.8'498—dc22

                                       2008046115

Contents

Foreword

> 66 **Where is the knowledge we have lost in information?** 99

—T.S. Eliot, "The Rock."

As modern civilization continues to evolve, its ability to create, store, distribute, and access information expands exponentially. The explosion of information from all media continues to increase at a phenomenal rate. By 2020 some experts predict the worldwide information base will double every 73 days. While access to diverse sources of information and perspectives is paramount to any democratic society, information alone cannot help people gain knowledge and understanding. Information must be organized and presented clearly and succinctly in order to be understood. The challenge in the digital age becomes not the creation of information, but how best to sort, organize, enhance, and present information.

ReferencePoint Press developed the *Compact Research* series with this challenge of the information age in mind. More than any other subject area today, researching current issues can yield vast, diverse, and unqualified information that can be intimidating and overwhelming for even the most advanced and motivated researcher. The *Compact Research* series offers a compact, relevant, intelligent, and conveniently organized collection of information covering a variety of current topics ranging from illegal immigration and deforestation to diseases such as anorexia and meningitis.

The series focuses on three types of information: objective single-author narratives, opinion-based primary source quotations, and facts and statistics. The clearly written objective narratives provide context and reliable background information. Primary source quotes are carefully selected and cited, exposing the reader to differing points of view. And facts and statistics sections aid the reader in evaluating perspectives. Presenting these key types of information creates a richer, more balanced learning experience.

For better understanding and convenience, the series enhances information by organizing it into narrower topics and adding design features that make it easy for a reader to identify desired content. For example, in *Compact Research: Illegal Immigration*, a chapter covering the economic impact of illegal immigration has an objective narrative explaining the various ways the economy is impacted, a balanced section of numerous primary source quotes on the topic, followed by facts and full-color illustrations to encourage evaluation of contrasting perspectives.

The ancient Roman philosopher Lucius Annaeus Seneca wrote, "It is quality rather than quantity that matters." More than just a collection of content, the *Compact Research* series is simply committed to creating, finding, organizing, and presenting the most relevant and appropriate amount of information on a current topic in a user-friendly style that invites, intrigues, and fosters understanding.

Sleep Disorders at a Glance

What Are Sleep Disorders?

A sleep disorder is any recurrent change in a normal sleep pattern. A sleep disorder can be as mild as insomnia or as serious as sleep apnea, narcolepsy, or sleepwalking, which can be potentially fatal disorders.

Prevalence

An estimated 70 million Americans suffer from sleep disorders, with the vast majority—60 million—suffering from chronic insomnia.

Causes

Most insomniacs eat late at night, watch TV in bed, drink too much coffee, or violate other rules of so-called good sleep hygiene. Many take their anxieties to bed with them. Other sleep disorder patients suffer from physical ailments that keep them up at night.

Diagnosis

Doctors monitor blood pressure, pulse, brain waves and breathing capacity to diagnose sleep apnea and hypersomnia. To diagnose restless legs syndrome, which causes insomnia, doctors will look for iron deficiencies and low red blood counts.

Costs to Society

Studies show that sleep disorders cost the American economy $20 billion a year or more in lost productivity and high health-care costs.

Severe Consequences

Sleep apnea can be fatal, cutting off air to the patient as he or she sleeps. Narcolepsy can be fatal if the patient falls asleep while driving. Insomniacs can also be responsible for fatal car accidents—drowsy driving causes some 1,500 deaths and 76,000 injuries a year.

Treatment

The sleep medication business has blossomed into a $2.8 billion industry.

Ongoing Research

Scientists are constantly unearthing new truths about sleep disorders, but there is still much they do not understand.

Overview

❝ The first thing to go is your sense of humor. Then goes the desire to do the things you used to do, then the desire to do anything at all. Parts of your body ache that you don't even know the names of, and your eyes forget how to focus.❞

—Gayle Greene, insomnia patient and author of *Insomniac.*

Any recurrent change in a normal sleep pattern is regarded as a sleep disorder. Sleep disorders range from insomnia, which is the inability to fall asleep, to some potentially serious illnesses that can lead to fatal complications such as sleep apnea, which makes it difficult to draw breaths while asleep, and narcolepsy, a sudden and unexpected fall into a deep sleep. People who suffer from sleep apnea can suffocate in their sleep. A narcoleptic who is driving a car can easily fall asleep at the wheel.

Still, most people who suffer from sleep disorders are insomniacs. Awake night after night, they watch the minutes tick off their bedside clocks, wondering whether they will ever fall asleep. Most of them eventually do catch a few hours of sleep, but not enough. The next morning they may feel cranky and unable to concentrate on their work or school. Says University of Chicago sleep expert Eve Van Cauter, "With lack of sleep, you're more likely to have a lower mood, less energy, more irritability."[1]

Everybody has nights when they cannot seem to fall asleep, but that does not mean they suffer from sleep disorders. Occasional sleeplessness can be attributed to many causes: a cup of coffee too close to bedtime, a problem pressing on the mind, a noisy neighbor. When the condition becomes chronic, only then can the patient be diagnosed with a sleep disorder. "Staying up late to watch TV is not insomnia," says Thomas Roth, director of the Sleep Disorders Research Center at Henry Ford Hospital in Detroit, Michigan. "But if you finish whatever you're doing, go to bed, and still can't sleep, that's insomnia—it's difficulty sleeping despite adequate opportunity."[2]

Two Categories

There are two categories of sleep disorders. The first category is dyssomnia, which results in poor sleep. Insomnia falls under this category, as does sleep apnea and narcolepsy. Other forms of dyssomnia are hypersomnia, which is a desire to sleep too much, and circadian rhythm disorders, an inability to maintain a regular sleep schedule. Night shift workers often suffer from circadian rhythm disorders.

Dyssomnia can be caused by external factors such as stress and anxiety. Also, dyssomnia can be caused by physiological factors such as obstructed breathing passageways, which can result in sleep apnea.

The other category is parasomnia, in which a part of the patient's brain wakes up even though the patient is still very much asleep. Parasomnia can prompt a sleeping patient into unusual and sometimes bizarre behaviors, such as sleep terrors, sleepwalking, or physical responses to nightmares, even though the patient will remember none of it when he or she wakes up.

> " Occasional sleeplessness can be attributed to many causes: a cup of coffee too close to bedtime, a problem pressing on the mind, a noisy neighbor. "

Other forms of parasomnia that are common in young children are bedwetting and head banging. Children who are head bangers slam their heads into their pillows for several minutes while they are asleep. Experts believe that head banging has a soothing and calming effect on young children—unconsciously, they desire the rocking motion of swaying their heads back and forth. Bed-wetting is attributed to a weak bladder in a child whose sleep is far deeper than that of a normal child—in other words, the bed wetter has to urinate more often than other children, and he or she is also more difficult to wake than others. Most children give up head banging and bed-wetting by the age of five.

Sleeplessness over the Ages

Sleep disorders first came to the attention of physicians during the era of the ancient Greeks. In the first century B.C., the Greek physician Heraclides recommended opium as a treatment for insomnia. William Shakespeare, who suffered from insomnia, afflicted many of his characters with an inability to sleep. Macbeth, for one, committed murder to seize the throne of Scotland and, haunted by his crime, endured insomnia. In Shakespeare's *Henry IV Part II*, the king observes that most of his subjects sleep soundly while he is kept awake by the pressures of his responsibilities:

> How many thousand of my poorest subjects
> Are at this hour asleep! O sleep, O gentle sleep,
> Nature's soft nurse, how have I frighted thee,
> That thou no more wilt weigh my eyelids down,
> And sleep my senses in forgetfulness?[3]

William Shakespeare, who suffered from insomnia, afflicted many of his characters with an inability to sleep. Macbeth, for one, committed murder to seize the throne of Scotland and, haunted by his crime, endured insomnia.

Over the centuries, most doctors were far more interested in how and why people dream than in how they sleep. The first published account of sleep apnea was not written by a doctor but by Charles Dickens, who described the sleep problems of an overweight boy named Joe in his 1836 novel *The Pickwick Papers*. For many years thereafter, sleep apnea was known as "Pickwickian syndrome."

Dickens knew something about sleep disorders because he suffered from insomnia himself. Other insomniacs of note include Winston Churchill, Napoléon Bonaparte, and the authors Marcel Proust and Alexander Dumas. And even though he claimed to know the benefits of going to bed early and rising early, Benjamin Franklin was also an insomniac.

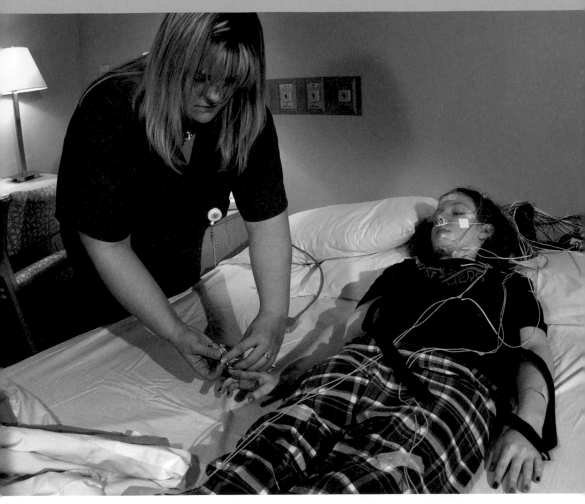

Cara, who is 16 years old, prepares to spend the night at the Sleep Disorders Center in Missouri. She is among a growing number of teenagers suffering from insomnia and other sleep disorders.

In 1913 French physician, Henri Piéron, published a study in which he suggested sleep problems could be attributed to physiological reasons, thereby establishing sleep disorders as physical illnesses. It was not until 1996, though, that the American Medical Association recognized sleep medicine as a specialty.

What Causes Sleeps Disorders?

Everybody experiences five stages of sleep, starting with stage 1, which is a transition between sleep and wakefulness. In stage 1, people experience light sleep; they will drift in and out of sleep and can easily be awakened. In stage 2, the electrical activity in the brain slows down. The heart rate also slows and body temperature dips. Stage 2 is also regarded as a period of light sleep. About half of a person's sleep is spent in stage 2.

> "In most cases, sleep disorders affect the ability of the patient to progress normally through the five stages of sleep.

In stages 3 and 4, which together are known as "slow-wave sleep," brain activity—known as brain waves—continues to slow. In these 2 stages, blood pressure and body temperature fall and breathing slows down. It is in stage 3 that the body becomes immobile. Stages 3 and 4 are regarded as deep sleep. People who are awakened during stages 3 or 4 are groggy and disoriented for several minutes after they wake up.

Stage 5 is known as rapid eye movement sleep, or REM sleep. It is known as REM sleep because the eyes move rapidly back and forth beneath the closed eyelids. During REM sleep, blood flow increases to the brain, the pulse quickens, and the breathing rate increases. REM sleep is the stage in which most people dream. During REM sleep, the body is paralyzed—evidently, a natural defense against the body acting out dreams. (The other four stages are also known as NREM sleep, for non–rapid eye movement sleep.)

About 20 percent of the sleeper's time is spent in REM sleep. Early in the sleep cycle, the REM stage will occur in short durations as the sleeper bounces between REM and the lighter stage of sleep. As dawn approaches, the REM periods will grow in length.

In most cases, sleep disorders affect the ability of the patient to progress normally through the five stages of sleep. In sleep apnea, for example, shortness of breath causes the patient to wake up many times over the course of the night. Since the patient is constantly waking and returning to sleep, he or she never reaches the deepest, most restful periods in the five stages. Says James O'Connor, director of the Sleep Disorders Center at Lancaster General Hospital in Pennsylvania, "We look to see whether people are getting the right amounts of each stage of sleep and whether someone stops breathing."[4]

Anxiety and Stress

When people take their problems to bed with them, it often results in a poor night's sleep. Indeed, anxiety and stress are regarded as primary reasons for insomnia. Actually, the body is wired to deal with stress, both physically and emotionally. When somebody is under stress, his or her brain responds by sending signals to the heart and other organs, telling them to prepare for trouble.

When someone is anxious or under stress, the heart will beat faster, blood pressure and body temperature will rise, and chemicals such as adrenaline and sugar will kick in, providing the body with energy to face the stressful situation. Of course, if it is the intention of the person to fall asleep at this time, then obviously the body's reaction to stress is not making it easy for sleep to occur.

Doctors call this condition hyper-arousal, meaning the body is in a highly aroused state and hardly in a condition conducive to sleep. Says author and insomnia patient Gayle Greene, "Insomniacs . . . have higher body temperature, faster heart rate and metabolism, because they are emotionally or cognitively aroused: they worry too much, they're upset, anxious or depressed, and . . . they have poor coping mechanisms."[5] Moreover, as many insomniacs lie awake at night, watching the shadows drift across the ceilings of their bedrooms, they grow even more anxious as they fret over another night of lost sleep.

> " When the circadian clock is running normally, the brain sends a signal to the body to be alert in the morning and drowsy at night. Obviously, people who work the night shift are getting the wrong signals from their internal clocks. "

Resetting the Internal Clock

Some sleep disorders can be attributed to direct physiological causes that can deprive the patient of restful sleep even if the patient feels no stress. For example, circadian rhythms can be disrupted by the amount of light that is absorbed by the brain through the eyes.

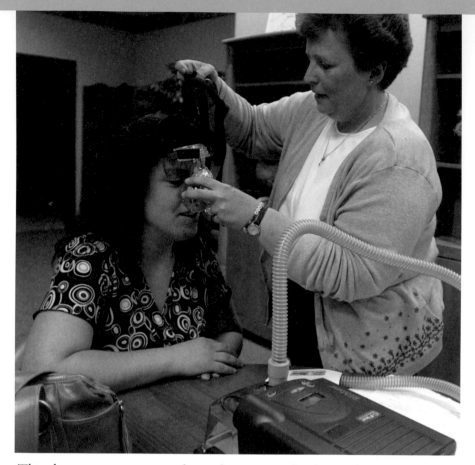

This sleep apnea patient is shown how to use the device that could cure her disorder. According to the Institute of Medicine sleep disorders affect an estimated 70 million Americans.

The eye contains millions of cells known as rods and cones. Their function is to collect light that passes through the lens of the eye, then transmit the light to the brain. That is how the brain forms an image of what the eye sees. Some of these rod and cone cells have another function—to gather light that is used by the brain to set the body's internal clock so that the body knows when it is day and night.

"Just like the ear has two functions—one is hearing and the other is balance—the eye has two functions," says Charles Czeisler, chief of sleep medicine at Brigham and Women's Hospital in Boston, Massachusetts. "One is this function of sight, so that we can see each other. And the other function is setting our internal clock so that we are awake during the daytime and able to sleep at night."[6]

When the circadian clock is running normally, the brain sends a signal to the body to be alert in the morning and drowsy at night. Obviously, people who work the night shift are getting the wrong signals from their internal clocks—they are receiving doses of the hormone melatonin, which induces sleep, as they show up for work, or their brains are telling them to be alert as they get ready for bed during daylight hours. That is why many night shift workers suffer from circadian rhythm disorders.

How Do Sleep Disorders Affect People?

Sleep is one of the fundamental processes of the body. It is as important to health as eating. Experts believe that every animal species on earth sleeps: dolphins sleep while swimming, horses sleep standing up, lions sleep for 12 hours a day, some bats sleep for months. As for people, most adults need 7 or 8 hours of sleep per day to feel fully rested. Teenagers need 9 hours. Babies require 16 hours a day.

The body repairs itself during sleep; studies have shown that cells produce more proteins during sleep, which enhances their growth. Says a publication of the National Sleep Foundation:

> " Insomnia can cause stress, anger, and irritability. People who do not sleep well may have trouble concentrating during the day. Their short-term memories may be impaired. "

> Although we naturally think of sleep as a time of rest and recovery from the stresses of everyday life, research is revealing that sleep is a dynamic activity, during which many processes vital to health and well-being take place. New evidence shows that sleep is essential to helping maintain mood, memory, and cognitive performance. It also plays a pivotal role in the normal function of the . . . immune system. In fact, studies show a growing link between sleep duration and a variety of serious health problems, including obesity, diabetes, hypertension, and depression.[7]

Indeed, sleep is essential to life—laboratory rats deprived of sleep have died. "It may not sound exciting," says neuroscientist Robert Vertes of Florida Atlantic University in Boca Raton, Florida, "but I think sleep is essential for rest."[8]

Consequences of Lack of Sleep

Insomnia can cause stress, anger, and irritability. People who do not sleep well may have trouble concentrating during the day. Their short-term memories may be impaired.

Moreover, lack of sleep can lead to illness. A study by the University of Chicago found that insomniacs produce less leptin, a hormone that tells the brain when the body is full, and more of the hormone ghrelin, which triggers hunger. In other words, insomniacs think they are hungry, and their brains are constantly telling them to keep eating. This heightens the risk of overeating, which can lead to obesity. "Chronic sleep deprivation causes changes in metabolism that produce a state that stimulates hunger,"[9] says Lawrence Epstein, medical director of the Sleep Health Centers in Boston.

People who do not sleep well are also at risk of developing depression. Studies have determined that people who do not sleep well produce high levels of cortisol, a hormone released during times of stress. The overproduction of this hormone increases the chance of being depressed. Depressed people are afflicted with feelings of sadness, hopelessness, and inadequacy. They lack the ability to enjoy life. "Positive moods are lower in people with sleep loss," says Van Cauter. "People have lower moods in the morning. They also have higher levels of cortisol, the stress hormone. All those changes are typical of clinical depression."[10]

The Tragedy of Reggie White

Reggie White played in the National Football League for 15 years. When he retired after the 2002 season, he was regarded as one of the best defensive linemen ever to have played professional football. Without question, he was headed for his sport's hall of fame.

But he had been plagued for years by sleep apnea—a common condition in obese or otherwise large men. (White weighed more than 300 pounds, or 136kg). One of the most familiar symptoms of sleep apnea is loud and robust snoring—a symptom that occurs as the sleeping patient tries to draw air into his or her lungs through a partially blocked airway. In White's case, his snoring seemed to shake the foundation of the family's home in Tennessee. His wife, Sara, insisted on going to bed before her husband so that she would be asleep before the snoring started.

On the morning of December 26, 2004, Sara White awoke to the sounds of her husband's snoring. "I pushed him over like I always did to get him to stop," she says. "I thought he was getting up, and then I realized he was coughing and choking." He then passed out. She said, "All I could think of was: 'How long has he been without oxygen?'"[11] Sara White called for an ambulance, but the paramedics could not revive her husband. The medical examiner later ruled that White's sleep apnea had helped trigger a fatal heart attack.

> Trucking companies, railroads, hospitals, and airlines—industries in which fatigued employees could put themselves and others in danger—have been among the leaders in providing facilities for workers to take naps when they feel they need a rest.

Can People Overcome Sleep Disorders?

For many people, the secret to getting a good night's sleep can be found in their mattresses. People have been sleeping on beds for some 10,000 years. Over time, the mattress has evolved from a fabric bag filled with straw or wool to today's mattresses, which provide support through a network of inner springs or, in some newer designs, beds of rubbery foam and air.

In the meantime, the sleeping pill and other sleeping medications have evolved over the years. In the nineteenth century, people took laudanum to help induce sleep. Laudanum was widely available as a patent medicine. Since the drug is made by mixing alcohol with opium, it had a strong effect. It was also highly addictive. In 1906 Congress passed the U.S. Pure Food and Drug Act, which led to the end of the patent medicine trade in America and, along with it, the use of laudanum as a sleep aid.

During the twentieth century, barbiturates gained widespread use as sleeping pills. Psychiatrists had been dispensing them to their patients to help reduce their anxieties. Barbiturates depress the body's central nervous system. They slow breathing and reduce the heart rate and blood pressure. They also tend to make people drowsy, so doctors frequently prescribed them as sleeping aids. Barbiturates could also be addictive, which is why doctors tend not to prescribe them to their insomnia patients today. Over the past decade, newer drugs have been developed that are believed to be very effective in inducing sleep. They are also regarded as less habit-forming than barbiturates.

Today the business of providing mattresses, drugs, and other aids to sleep-deprived people has blossomed into a $20 billion a year industry. Says Peter Bils, an executive with the mattress company Select Comfort, "We firmly believe—no pun intended—that a mattress can make significant changes in sleep quality."[12]

Sleeping on the Job

In 1902 the Barcolo Manufacturing Company of Buffalo, New York, established its place in American business history by becoming the first corporation to offer its employees coffee breaks. The employees of the furniture company had asked executives for 15-minute breaks in the midmorning and midafternoon. Instead of finding production slowing because of the two daily work stoppages, the Barcolo executives were pleasantly surprised to find production actually increased. The reason? The caffeine-rich coffee consumed by the employees provided them with a jolt of energy. Soon businesses throughout America were offering coffee breaks to their workers.

" Sleep experts also advise people to leave their anxieties and worries outside their bedrooms. "

Today some companies have developed far different attitudes about the welfare of their workers. They have acknowledged the dangers of fatigued employees and encourage their workers to take brief naps on company time, and they have even outfitted their offices with lounge furniture. Trucking companies, railroads, hospitals, and airlines—industries in which fatigued employees could put themselves and others in danger—have been among the leaders in providing facilities for workers to take naps when they feel they need a rest. Other companies have gotten the message as well. At Yarde Metals in Pelham, New Hampshire, the company has provided a room of "nap pods"—lounge chairs outfitted with lightproof and soundproof domes. Says Yarde Metals branch manager Steve Rogers, "It's an opportunity for [employees] if they need a refresher to take a quick nap in peace and quiet and get back to work."[13]

"Peace of Mind"

Sleep experts agree that there is no magic solution for insomniacs or others who suffer from sleep disorders. For insomniacs, their best hope is to make use of the therapies available—drugs if they need them, but they should also maintain healthy lifestyles and good "sleep hygiene."

Sleep hygiene is what doctors call the conditions under which people try to sleep. They urge people to maintain regular sleep schedules and not allow themselves to sleep late on weekends. Their bedrooms should be cool, dark, and uncluttered. They should not use the bed for purposes other than sleep—no eating or watching TV in bed. Sleep experts urge people to avoid eating within three hours of bedtime and stay away from coffee and other caffeinated beverages in the evening.

Sleep experts also advise people to leave their anxieties and worries outside their bedrooms. They point out that a century or more ago, most people had to share beds with other members of their families. They may have had to endure the snoring of their parents and the blanket hogging of their younger siblings. Their bedrooms were probably heated by fireplaces, which certainly died down overnight, leaving the rooms as cold as the frigid outdoors. Bedbugs and other vermin may have been living in the mattresses. On the floor by the bed rested a smelly chamber pot.

But if people could leave their troubles at the door, chances are they probably got a good night's sleep. Says James Horne, director of sleep research at Loughborough University in England, "It's peace of mind rather than physical comfort that counts, anyway."[14]

What Are Sleep Disorders?

66 Recently I began to snore. And not just your cute little snore, mind you. This was loud enough to cause my wife to vibrate next to me in bed and to disturb the kids in the next room. Got the picture? My wife, after being awakened on numerous occasions, became really concerned when she noted that during my sleep I had severe episodes of choking and gasping. 99

—Ralph E. Dittman, a sleep apnea patient and research scientist at Baylor College of Medicine in Houston, Texas.

More than 70 million Americans, nearly a quarter of the U.S. population, are believed to suffer from sleep disorders. The sleep disorder that afflicts the most people is insomnia—some 60 million Americans suffer from the inability to consistently get restful sleep. That total does not even count the number of Americans who do not fit the clinical description of insomnia but nevertheless insist that they are dissatisfied with their sleep. According to a 2008 poll by the National Sleep Foundation, 62 percent of the respondents said they get a good night's sleep a few nights a month only.

In simple terms, insomnia is the inability to fall asleep or stay asleep. Indeed, insomniacs who do manage to fall asleep spend very little time in stages of deep sleep; mostly they drift between wakefulness and sleep stages 1 and 2. They may wake up several times a night or wake up early in the morning, hours before their alarms are set to go off, and find themselves unable to get back to sleep. Since they spend little or no time in the deep sleep stages, they never feel rested the next morning.

Gayle Greene, an author and college professor, says she has lived with insomnia since childhood. Despite trying all manner of medications and other therapies and changing her daily routine, sleep hygiene, and lifestyle, she is still unable to sleep for more than two or three hours a night. And after each fitful night, she faces a day of sluggishness, irritability, and an inability to concentrate. Says Greene:

> When you get out of bed, brain like a fried sponge, mood like something left out of the refrigerator too long, bad luck, just write it off, just hope that the sleep fairy drops by the next night . . . but meanwhile, there's this day to live through, this whole long day. . . .
>
> They call this a "sleep disorder," but it's actually an all-day disorder. Insomnia is not just something that happens to the night; it happens to the day, the whole of the day, and if it's chronic insomnia, it happens to many days. A half-life of ruined days.[15]

Narcolepsy: Paralyzing Sleep

Narcolepsy causes people to fall asleep suddenly. The disorder afflicts about 1 in 2,000 people. Narcolepsy can be a particularly dangerous affliction if the patient is driving a car or operating heavy machinery when hit by a narcoleptic episode.

Narcolepsy is not the body's reaction to insomnia: In other words, narcoleptics do not fall asleep during the day because they failed to get a restful sleep the night before. People who sleep soundly all night can suffer from narcolepsy.

Narcoleptics can fall asleep anywhere and at any time. They may be carrying on a conversation with friends when they suddenly nod off. Many narcoleptics also suffer from cataplexy, a condition in which the muscles suddenly go weak. Speech may also become slurred during a cataplexic episode. In most cases, cataplexy will last for a few seconds or minutes.

> " More than 70 million Americans, nearly a quarter of the U.S. population, are believed to suffer from sleep disorders. "

Narcoleptics can also suffer from sleep paralysis. For a few seconds or minutes prior to falling asleep, they can become paralyzed—unable to move their arms, legs, or other parts of their bodies. At this point, they have not yet fallen asleep, so they are well aware that they have lapsed into a paralyzed state. It can be a frightening experience.

> In sleep apnea, the blockage in the patient's throat causes breathing to become very shallow or even to stop for periods of 10 or 20 seconds.

Tim Costa, a professional bass fisherman from Catskill, New York, suffered his first narcoleptic attack in 2005 while grocery shopping. Reaching into a freezer to pick up a bag of frozen chicken, Costa suddenly felt the freezer's coldness overwhelm his body. Paralyzed, Costa collapsed to the floor. He was unable to talk but could see and hear the customers and store employees gathering around him. He recovered from the cataplexic episode after a few minutes but soon found himself a victim of full-blown narcolepsy, falling asleep once or twice a day. "It was a toxic kind of tiredness," he says. "It consumes you. Imagine being so exhausted your whole body feels like pins and needles. Your arms and legs feel long and heavy. I just had to go sit down and let it happen."[16]

Hypersomnia: "Impossible to Stay Awake"

Hypersomniacs fall into deep sleeps and cannot easily be roused. They may sleep 16 or 20 hours a day. Hypersomnia is often a symptom of depression and other mental illnesses—patients cannot summon the energy to get out of bed. Or, if they do rise from their beds in the morning, it is likely they will take naps during the day. Unlike insomniacs, hypersomniacs can easily lapse into the deep sleep stages.

There are two types of hypersomnia: idiopathic and traumatic. In idiopathic hypersomnia, physicians are unable to determine the cause, while the cause of traumatic hypersomnia can usually be traced to brain injuries, drug or alcohol abuse, side effects from medication, or similar external events. Experts believe that 1 in 20,000 people suffer from idiopathic hypersomnia.

British patient Anne Wollenberg, 27, has been afflicted with hypersomnia since she was a teenager. According to Wollenberg, she has no difficulty sleeping through blaring alarm clocks. "I slept deeply as a child," Wollenberg says. "Chronic drowsiness hit when I reached adolescence—I had trouble waking up, was often late for school and sometimes fell asleep during lessons. My concentration levels were poor and I had no energy."[17]

Eventually, Wollenberg was diagnosed with idiopathic hypersomnia. At a sleep clinic, she was tested by being asked to take naps under the observation of nurses and physicians. Wollenberg thought it would be impossible to fall asleep under such circumstances, but instead she quickly drifted into deep stages of sleep each time she was tested. Says Wollenberg, "I thought it would be difficult to keep falling asleep in a strange place with people observing, but instead found it almost impossible to stay awake."[18]

Sleep Apnea: A Killer

Sleep apnea is caused by blocked air passages mostly affecting obese or otherwise large men, but others, including women, are susceptible as well. (In Greek, *apnea* means "without breath.") Even otherwise healthy toddlers have been diagnosed with obstructive sleep apnea, meaning the airways leading to their lungs are partially blocked during sleep. Indeed, parents of very young sleep apnea patients are often puzzled when their children start snoring. "People used to think snoring in children wasn't a problem, it was just cute," says Stuart Tomares, director of the Pediatric Sleep Center at Suburban Hospital in Bethesda, Maryland. "But it's not cute. It can be indicative of a serious disorder."[19] An estimated 2 percent of adult women and 4 percent of adult men suffer from sleep apnea. In addition, as many as 3 percent of American children may also suffer from symptoms of apnea.

> " Patients who suffer from circadian rhythm disorders cannot coordinate their sleeping habits with their inner biological clocks, which are telling them when it is daytime and nighttime. "

Among the complications caused by sleep apnea are high blood pressure and heart disease. In sleep apnea, the blockage in the patient's throat causes breathing to become very shallow or even to stop for periods of 10 or 20 seconds. When breathing is interrupted, the patient responds by waking up—then falling right back to sleep. It is not unusual for a sleep apnea patient to wake up and fall asleep hundreds of times a night. But the patient is not aware that his or her breathing has been interrupted. Of course, since the patient is constantly waking up and going back to sleep, he or she does not enter the deepest stages of sleeping. As a result, the next day the patient is not well rested. Indeed, sleep apnea patients tend to nod off during the day.

A 2007 study conducted by the New Jersey–based Living Heart Foundation found that 75 percent of retired NFL linemen suffer from sleep apnea. Says Allan Levy, team physician for the New York Giants:

> The problem with sleep apnea is the neck. A 17½-inch neck is usually where the problem begins. The muscles relax in the body. Now the weight of the neck clasps down on their airways. They stop breathing. They momentarily wake up, then the cycle starts over again, and they never get into deep sleep. They develop heart disease and hypertension. Sleep apnea is a killer. One of the kids that played for us, we did a sleep study on, had 440 awakenings during the night.[20]

Circadian Rhythm Disorders

Patients who suffer from circadian rhythm disorders cannot coordinate their sleeping habits with their inner biological clocks, which are telling them when it is daytime and nighttime. In other words, their brains are not in sync with the normal daytime-nighttime routine of sleeping and rising. Jet lag is the most common form—travelers who cross many time zones may find themselves weary and ready for bed even though the sun is rising as their planes touch down. When they get to their hotel rooms they may drop off into deep sleeps, but when night arrives they may not be able to get to sleep because they have done their sleeping during the day.

"Most processes within our bodies are regulated by a 24-hour timing mechanism or clock that can be called our 'biological clock,'" says Chris Colwell, a psychiatry professor at the University of California–Los Angeles. "Rapid travel between time zones temporarily disrupts this biological clock and results in the set of symptoms known as jet lag. Our system does readjust but it takes time. It can take a couple of weeks to adjust to the new time in Europe or Asia."[21]

Indeed, travelers eventually adjust to their new time zones and most will be able to sleep on normal schedules, but night shift workers face a nightly conflict with their circadian clocks. People whose jobs require them to work overnight are constantly told by their brains that they should be getting to bed as they arrive for work. In fact, in the evening, the brain releases the hormone melatonin, which enhances people's abilities to fall asleep. This is the brain's way of telling the body that it is time for bed. There are some 15 million night shift workers in America—it is likely that many of them endure a nightly battle against their own circadian clocks.

Nightmare Disorder: Reliving Terrifying Ordeals

Everybody has nightmares from time to time—as with most dreams, they tend to occur during REM sleep—but 5 percent of the population is believed to suffer from nightmare disorder, meaning their nightmares are regular and recurring. When they have nightmares, they often wake up in terror with a racing pulse, breathing heavily and drenched in sweat. Since REM sleep is most elongated in the hours before dawn, that is when nightmare disorders typically occur.

Many post-traumatic stress disorder patients suffer from nightmare disorders. These patients are often former members of the military who have been affected emotionally by warfare. Victims of crime are often afflicted with post-traumatic stress disorder. They find themselves reliving the terrifying circumstances that led to their disorder, often in their dreams.

> " People who suffer from sleep terrors have a physical reaction to nightmares: They will sit up in bed, screaming or crying. "

Others who may be afflicted with nightmare disorders are people who are depressed, as well as people who feel vulnerable in some way. Psychiatrists have found that nightmare disorders plague people whose conscious thoughts and daydreams are often vivid and disturbing. "Nightmares can have many influences, but for these people nightmares are a bad habit," says Barry

Krakow, director of the Center for Sleep Medicine and Nightmare Treatment in Albuquerque, New Mexico. "They're a learned behavior."[22]

Sleep Terrors: Frightening Young Children

Sleep terrors, also known as night terrors, afflict mostly children, but some adults suffer from the disorder. People who suffer from sleep terrors have a physical reaction to nightmares: They will sit up in bed, screaming or crying. As with nightmare disorder patients, they will have a racing pulse and rapid breathing. Their muscles will be tense, as though they are poised for action. They may wear confused looks on their faces. However, they are still asleep, which means their parents or spouses cannot give them comfort. In the morning, they remember nothing of their ordeals.

> "Sleepwalkers have been lampooned for decades on TV and in the movies, but there is little about the affliction that would suggest it should rightly be a topic for humor.

"Night terrors usually occur about two hours after a child falls asleep, when the first cycle of deep sleep has suddenly come to an end and light waking has not fully occurred,"[23] says Joshua D. Sparrow, a pediatric psychiatrist at Harvard University Medical School in Massachusetts.

Experts believe that sleep terrors patients are feeling anxious. It is estimated that some 200,000 children experience sleep terrors to some degree each year. In the case of young children, doctors urge their parents to be especially soothing at bedtime.

Sleepwalking: Dangerous Behavior

Sleepwalkers have been lampooned for decades on TV and in the movies, but there is little about the affliction that would suggest it should rightly be a topic for humor. The experiences of Canadian tennis star Peter Polansky show that sleepwalking—its medical term is somnambulism—is a serious disorder that can lead to injury or even death.

In 2006 Polansky, 17, arrived in Mexico City to participate in a tournament. One night Polansky experienced an episode of sleepwalking, stepping out of his hotel window and plummeting three floors. Luckily, his fall was broken by some shrubbery below. He survived the fall, although he sustained a serious gash to his leg, which was cut by broken glass from the window.

Polansky said he had been dreaming and believed an intruder entered his room with a knife. In response, he jumped out of bed and kicked out the window to escape. "I remember kicking the bottom window and the next thing I know I was on my back," he says. "I saw my leg totally cut open."[24]

As many as 4 percent of American adults are believed to suffer from somnambulism to some degree. As the name of the disorder suggests, sleepwalkers carry out physical acts while still asleep—in most cases, they will get out of bed and move around the house. Since they are asleep, they do not respond to others. Many will return to bed before waking up. Like sleep terrors, sleepwalking afflicts mostly young children, but many people are plagued by sleepwalking episodes into their adult years. "It's dangerous behavior," says Harvey Moldofsky, director of the Sleep Disorders Clinic at the University of Toronto. "Usually, these people in a sleep terror are overwhelmed with intense fear and it's a very primitive type of response—fight or flight."[25]

Many people endure sleep disorders. They may be perfectly healthy in all other respects, but for reasons they cannot explain, they cannot seem to fall asleep at night or stay awake during the day. Others risk serious injury: narcoleptics, who can fall asleep while driving a car; sleep apnea sufferers, who could suffocate at night; or sleepwalkers, who can do harm to themselves when they come to believe in their sleepy minds that they are no longer safe in their own beds.

Primary Source Quotes*

What Are Sleep Disorders?

66 I am really very tired of being told what it's like to live in my body by people who haven't a clue. I have come to feel that, when it comes to insomnia, there is truth to the old adage, it takes one to know one. 99

—Gayle Greene, *Insomniac*. Berkeley and Los Angeles: University of California Press, 2008.

Greene, a professor of literature at Scripps College in Claremont, California, is an insomnia patient and author of the book *Insomniac*.

66 There's definitely this cyclical nature that goes on where you don't get a lot of sleep and that triggers a low mood. And then when you have a low mood, it makes your sleep worse, and the two sort of feed off each other. 99

—Todd Arnedt, in Neal Conan, "Insomnia Keeps 60 Million Americans Up at Night," *Talk of the Nation*, National Public Radio, April 20, 2008.

Arnedt is fellowship director of the Sleep Disorder Center at the University of Michigan.

* Editor's Note: While the definition of a primary source can be narrowly or broadly defined, for the purposes of Compact Research, a primary source consists of: 1) results of original research presented by an organization or researcher; 2) eyewitness accounts of events, personal experience, or work experience; 3) first-person editorials offering pundits' opinions; 4) government officials presenting political plans and/or policies; 5) representatives of organizations presenting testimony or policy.

"You don't remember falling asleep and you don't remember waking up. That's really hard on a person."

—Tim Costa, in Cathleen F. Crowley, "Sleep Deprived: A Tired Fisherman Learns His Exhaustion Is Tied to Disorders," *Albany Times Union*, September 25, 2007.

Costa is a narcolepsy patient and professional bass fisherman who lives in Catskill, New York.

"The primary treatment for sleep apnea is to lose weight and they can't. There's no such thing as a 225-pound offensive lineman. We try to make certain that they understand that they've got to come down in weight when they retire."

—Allan Levy, in Clifton Brown, "Ex-Players Dealing with Not-So-Glamorous Health Issues," *New York Times*, February 1, 2007.

Levy is a team physician for the New York Giants.

"I wasn't even snoring. I just wasn't breathing for a whole minute and that was scary when I found out. I always wondered why I needed to drink two to three cups of coffee and Red Bull during the day."

—Vicente Solano, in Miriam Ramirez, "Affecting 1 in 5 Americans, Sleep Apnea Can Prove Fatal to Sufferers," *McAllen (TX) Monitor*, November 27, 2006.

Solano, a sleep apnea patient, lives in McAllen, Texas.

---

66 In sleep apnea, the brain has to awaken the sufferer in order for breathing to start again. Frequent arousals from apneic events during the night prevent the person from getting enough deep, restorative sleep. **99**

—National Sleep Foundation, *Sleep-Wake Cycle: Its Physiology and Impact on Health*, 2006.

The National Sleep Foundation supports research into sleep disorders and provides information to the public as well as training for health-care providers on sleep disorders.

66 Nothing in evolution prepared us for jet travel or jet lag. **99**

—Charles Weitz, in Dan Vergano, "Your Body's on the Clock with Circadian Rhythms," *USA Today*, June 19, 2007.

Weitz is professor of neurobiology at Harvard University Medical School in Massachusetts.

66 The more deep sleep you have, the more likely you are to have a night terror or sleepwalk. That's another reason why this is more common in kids. Kids spend a greater percentage of their sleep time in deep sleep than adults do. **99**

—Judy Owens, in Debbe Geiger, "'Night-Night' Holds Peril, Sleepwalking and Night Terrors: Unsettling but Normal Childhood Stages," *Newsday*, March 7, 2006.

Owens is director of the Pediatric Sleep Disorders Clinic at Hasbro Children's Hospital in Providence, Rhode Island.

" Night terrors . . . are [a] different kind of sleep phenomenon. They are more frequent in childhood. They usually don't have any specific imagery involved, but they have this sort of terrifying, physically convulsing effect. "

—Kelly Bulkeley, in Neal Conan, "The Science Behind Dreams and Nightmares," *Talk of the Nation*, National Public Radio, October 30, 2007.

Bulkeley is a member of the faculty of the Dream Studies Program at John F. Kennedy University in California.

" They're scary to watch. He would look right at you, but he'd be flailing and screaming, and he had no idea I was there. It's almost like watching a zombie. He'd never remember anything the next day. "

—Marie Silver, in Debbe Geiger, "'Night-Night' Holds Peril, Sleepwalking and Night Terrors: Unsettling but Normal Childhood Stages," *Newsday*, March 7, 2006.

Silver, of Massapequa, New York, is the mother of a two-year-old boy, Garrett, who experiences frequent sleep terrors.

What Are Sleep Disorders?

- At least **70 million** Americans suffer from sleep disorders, including **60 million** who are afflicted with insomnia.

- **Eighty percent** of American teenagers sleep less than the recommended nine hours per night.

- **Sixty-five percent** of Americans report having problems falling asleep at least a few nights per month; **44 percent** say they have problems falling asleep either every night or nearly every night.

- A Texas study found that **25 percent** of teenagers have trouble falling asleep and staying asleep; **5 percent** of teenagers say their insomnia affects their daytime activities.

- Obstructive sleep apnea affects **2 percent** of adult women and **4 percent** of adult men.

- A study published in the *New England Journal of Medicine* found that **14 percent** of active NFL players suffer from sleep apnea.

- **Twenty-nine percent** of Americans say they wake up before their alarms go off and cannot fall back asleep.

- As many as **12 percent** of young children snore, while **2 to 3 percent** of young children suffer from obstructive sleep apnea.

- As many as **17 percent** of children have walked in their sleep; in adults, nearly **4 percent** are believed to be sleepwalkers.

- Sleep terrors affect as many as **3 percent** of adults.

Many People Have Problems Sleeping

The National Sleep Foundation queried 1,000 Americans on their sleeping habits and learned that 44 percent suffer from insomnia or other sleep disorders on a nightly or near nightly basis. About a quarter of the respondents wake up during the night while more than 10 percent say they wake up too early and can't fall back to sleep. Other respondents say they suffer from sleep disorders on an occasional basis. A small minority of respondents say they sleep very well every night.

Frequency of Sleep Problem in Last Month

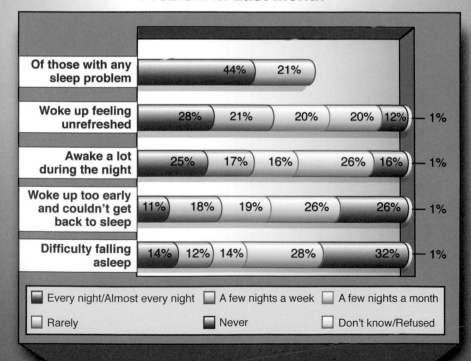

	Every night/Almost every night	A few nights a week	A few nights a month	Rarely	Never	Don't know/Refused
Of those with any sleep problem	44%	21%				
Woke up feeling unrefreshed	28%	21%	20%	20%	12%	1%
Awake a lot during the night	25%	17%	16%	26%	16%	1%
Woke up too early and couldn't get back to sleep	11%	18%	19%	26%	26%	1%
Difficulty falling asleep	14%	12%	14%	28%	32%	1%

Source: National Sleep Foundation, *2008 Sleep in American Poll*, 2008. www.sleepfoundation.org.

Sleep Disorders in Children

Researchers assessed the sleeping habits of 494 children in kindergarten through the fourth grade and found many suffer from insomnia, sleep terrors, nightmare disorders, and sleepwalking. More than 18 percent of the children snore loudly while about 4 percent of the children snort and gasp in their sleep, which indicates that they are on their way to developing sleep apnea. Most of the children suffer from insomnia: More than 15 percent are unable to fall asleep within 20 minutes while nearly 20 percent do not get enough sleep.

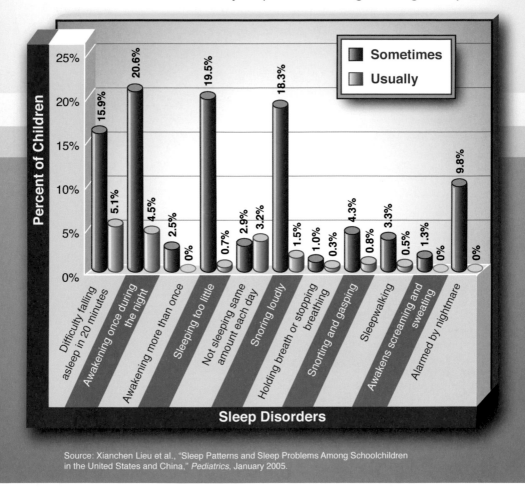

Source: Xianchen Lieu et al., "Sleep Patterns and Sleep Problems Among Schoolchildren in the United States and China," *Pediatrics*, January 2005.

- **Forty-nine percent** of Americans say they do not wake up in the morning feeling refreshed.

Many Adults Discuss Sleep Problems with Their Doctor

A study by the U.S. Centers for Disease Control and Prevention found that nearly 30 percent of American adults tell their doctors that they have trouble sleeping. Statistics show that women are more likely to complain about sleep problems to their doctors, but men, by a slight margin, are more likely to be diagnosed with sleep apnea.

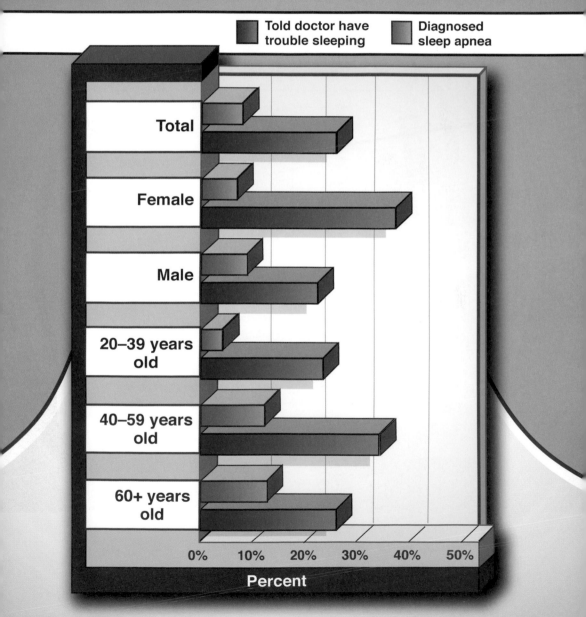

Legend:
- Told doctor have trouble sleeping
- Diagnosed sleep apnea

Categories (top to bottom): Total, Female, Male, 20–39 years old, 40–59 years old, 60+ years old

X-axis: Percent — 0%, 10%, 20%, 30%, 40%, 50%

Source: Edward J. Sondik, National Center for Health Statistics, U.S. Centers for Disease Control and Prevention, *Healthy People 2010*, May 22, 2008. www.cdc.gov.

People Who Sleep Too Much

Unlike insomnia patients, people who suffer from idiopathic hypersomnia (excessive sleeping with prolonged sleep episodes) and narcolepsy sleep too much. A study by British researchers looked at some of the characteristics of hypersomnia and narcolepsy patients, and found that the symptoms of hypersomnia start manifesting themselves in adolescence while most narcoleptics first start experiencing the symptoms of the disorder in early adulthood. Also, the study revealed that narcoleptics and hypersomniacs typically wait many years before they talk to their doctors. A total of 77 hypersomniac and 63 narcoleptic patients participated in the study. Not surprisingly, more than half of the hypersomnia patients had trouble getting out of bed, which is one of the main symptoms of the disorder.

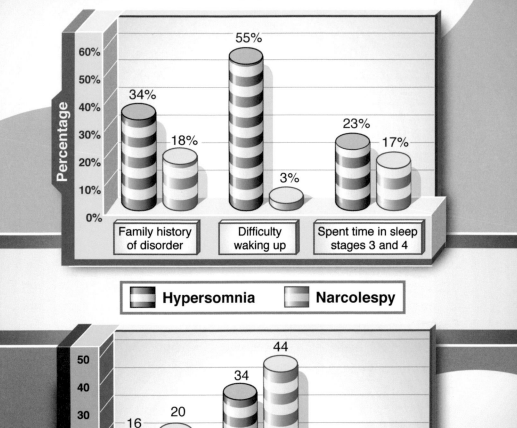

Source: Kirstie M. Anderson et al., "Idiopathic Hypersomnia: A Study of 77 Cases," *Sleep*, October 1, 2007.

What Causes Sleep Disorders?

> **The word *nightwalkers* describes people (like me) who are forced to endure profoundly disagreeable creepy-crawly symptoms in their legs that can be relieved only by movement or medication. Walking is the method most commonly used, and since the restless limbs suffer more at night, the severely afflicted may have to walk all night long.**

—Robert H. Yoakum, author and restless legs syndrome patient.

A nxiety, stress, emotional problems, and poor sleep hygiene all contribute to insomnia as well as other sleep disorders, but for many years doctors have believed that physiological problems can also contribute to poor sleep. Research has revealed that many sleep disorders are caused by chemical imbalances in the brain and body. For example, an interruption in the flow of the hormone melatonin can make it difficult for some people to fall asleep while narcoleptics suffer from a lack of the hormone hypocretin in their bodies. Hypocretin provides the body with a boost of energy; people who lack a sufficient quantity of the hormone will have trouble staying awake.

Physiological reasons are often at the root of sleep apnea—obstructions in the human airway that occur naturally in the throat may inhibit people's abilities to draw breaths while they sleep. Abnormalities in other parts of the body may also cause sleeplessness: New evidence continues to surface suggesting that a restless mind may not be the only cause of insomnia—restless legs may also be keeping people up at night.

Restless Legs Syndrome

As late as the 1990s, restless legs syndrome, or RLS, was still an obscure disorder that puzzled many doctors when their patients complained that prickly and uncomfortable twitches and other sensations in their legs were keeping them awake at night. Now doctors have a much better understanding of the affliction. It is also known as nightwalking or Ekbom's syndrome, after Swedish neurologist Karl A. Ekbom, who first wrote about the syndrome in 1945. As physicians have become more familiar with the symptoms of RLS, they have been more willing to diagnose it. Now it is believed that a staggering 10 percent of the American population may suffer from restless legs syndrome, although far fewer people, about 3 percent, suffer the affliction to a degree that may require treatment.

Sherry Dagnall, 44, wrestled with the affliction for many years without knowing why her legs felt so strange at night. RLS was not only keeping her up at night, it was keeping her husband up as well: She tossed and turned so much that neither was getting a good night's sleep. "I flopped all over the bed,"[26] she says. Finally, she was diagnosed with RLS.

At first, doctors believed RLS was caused by psychological reasons—that patients' anxieties manifested themselves in physical symptoms. Research has shown, though, that there may be a number of physical causes of RLS, including anemia, a condition in which patients suffer from deficiencies of red blood cells. An iron deficiency in the blood may also cause RLS. In addition, nerve damage caused by diabetes may contribute to RLS. About a quarter of all pregnant women suffer from RLS, perhaps because the baby presses against nerves or blood vessels, restricting blood flow to the legs. The condition usually clears up after women give birth. RLS is believed to be hereditary, meaning it runs in families and is, therefore, passed on from generation to generation.

A Life-Altering Ailment

About 80 percent of RLS patients experience periodic limb movements, which are regular and explosive jerks of their feet or legs that can jolt them awake. In addition, RLS can afflict patients during the day. Many patients cannot travel in airplanes or drive for long distances in cars. They cannot enjoy movies or concerts because the constant tingling sensation in their legs makes them want to get up and walk around. RLS patients who work in offices find they cannot sit at their desks for long. Many of them cannot sit through meetings. For many patients, RLS has altered their lives, forcing them to make decisions about changing their careers and lifestyles.

Peter Brooks had to give up his career as an investment banker because RLS kept him up at night and further tortured him during the day. "I had trouble sleeping and would wake up and have to walk around for hours," he says. "My job also involved a lot of travel and it became increasingly difficult to be strapped into an airplane seat for five hours or so."[27]

At the age of 50, Brooks quit his job in New York City and moved to Pebble Beach, California. He works as a professional artist, a job that gives him much more freedom of movement—he is not forced to sit behind a desk or travel.

Another RLS patient, Ed Murfin, a 69-year-old retired minister from Jacksonville, Florida, recalled suffering from RLS as a young boy and being made to stand in the corner by elementary school teachers because he fidgeted so much at his classroom desk. Humiliated so much by the way he was treated by his teachers and others who did not understand his ailment, Murfin eventually lapsed into a period of depression. "I had a breakdown that wiped out several years of my life,"[28] he says.

> " New evidence continues to surface suggesting that a restless mind may not be the only cause of insomnia—restless legs may also be keeping people up at night. "

Melatonin Deficiencies

Melatonin, the hormone that enhances people's ability to fall asleep, is suppressed if too much light is absorbed through the eyes. That is a main reason night shift workers suffer from circadian rhythm disorders—the ailment is triggered by the light transmitted from the eyes into the brain. Essentially, night shift workers are trying to get to bed at a time when the sun is rising and their eyes are absorbing the light of the new day. The process is called circadian photoreception.

Melatonin is manufactured and released from the pea-size pineal gland, which can be found in the center of the brain. Overnight, the pineal gland continues to release melatonin throughout slumber. As dawn approaches—and the sun rises, brightening people's bedrooms—the production of melatonin slows.

> Melatonin, the hormone that enhances people's ability to fall asleep, is suppressed if too much light is absorbed through the eyes.

Melatonin deficiencies also affect others who have trouble sleeping. In most people, the pineal gland starts releasing melatonin a few hours before bedtime. Melatonin may also have an effect on body temperature, lowering it as the hour of sleep approaches—a lower body temperature enhances the ability to fall asleep. In insomniacs, the pineal gland produces less melatonin than they need to fall asleep. Also, it has been proven that as people age, the amount of melatonin produced by their brains is reduced.

Another part of the brain that regulates sleep is the suprachiasmatic nucleus, or SCN, found in the hypothalamus, deep in the center of the brain. The SCN is the location of the circadian clock, which lets the body know when it is nighttime and daytime and, therefore, when it is time to go to bed and time to wake up. The circadian rhythms are constantly adjusting themselves as the days and nights grow longer or shorter according to the seasons.

Why Women Cannot Sleep

Bloating, soreness, cramps, headaches, and other symptoms of menstruation often interrupt women's sleep—a study by the National Sleep Foundation found that 70 percent of women report sleep problems for 2.5 days during their menstrual periods. Women who suffer from premenstrual syndrome, or PMS, also experience sleep problems. In PMS, women experience mood swings, irritability, changes in appetite, and tension—all factors that could keep them up at night. The National Sleep Foundation study found that 60 percent of PMS sufferers said they had trouble sleeping during their premenstrual episodes. Moreover, some of the PMS patients reported other sleep disorders, including hypersomnia and nightmare disorders. In addition, women who take birth control pills often find a side effect of the pills is a rise in body temperature—a factor that contributes to insomnia.

Older women who enter menopause—in which they undergo hormonal changes and stop menstruating—find themselves suffering from insomnia. About 80 percent of women entering menopause experience "hot flashes"—sudden increases in their body temperatures, which often occur at night, waking them up. Also, hot flashes can cause night sweats, soaking their bed clothes, then chilling them as they cool down. Says Gayle Greene: "At menopause, women's sleep complaints more than double. Hot flashes are the explanation given by most sleep experts—and, no doubt, hot flashes may disrupt sleep."[29]

The Kick of Caffeine

Caffeine is a chemical found in coffee beans, tea leaves, cacao beans (which are used to make chocolate), and kola nuts (which are used in the manufacture of cola soft drinks). Caffeine can be extracted from plants and used as an additive. Beverages such as Red Bull and Mountain Dew contain high concentrations of caffeine that are added artificially. Caffeine is a stimulant, meaning it makes people alert and gives them energy. Many people enjoy a cup of coffee at breakfast because it helps wake them up. People who drink several cups of coffee a day as well as other caffeinated beverages frequently have trouble sleeping.

Caffeine affects neurotransmitters, the chemicals that carry messages from brain cell to brain cell. Caffeine blocks the release of the neurotransmitter adenosine, which slows down the release of other neurotransmitters. When adenosine is allowed to flow normally, it slows down the electrical activity in the brain. People whose brains generate a lot of electrical activity—in other words, people who are constantly alert—often find it very difficult to fall asleep.

> **Many people enjoy a cup of coffee at breakfast because it helps wake them up. People who drink several cups of coffee a day as well as caffeinated beverages frequently have trouble sleeping.**

Moreover, when the brain is alert the body responds by releasing the hormone adrenaline. Adrenaline prepares the body for activity—it raises blood pressure and increases the heart rate. Adrenaline also helps pump blood into the muscles. At this point, the body is primed for action—perhaps a vigorous game of basketball, but certainly not sleep.

Caffeine increases the flow of the neurotransmitter dopamine. Dopamine enhances memory and attention—again, two mental states that are hardly conducive to falling asleep. Finally, caffeine suppresses the release of melatonin, perhaps the most vital chemical in the body when it comes to sleep. After caffeine is consumed, it will stay in the body for hours. This means that people who drink as little as two cups of coffee a day may have trouble falling asleep at night.

People who *do not* want to sleep—they may want to stay awake so they can study late into the night or work the night shift—may resort to drinking a lot of coffee. The nineteenth-century French author Honoré de Balzac preferred to work on his novels for days at a time with no breaks for sleep. To work under those conditions, Balzac consumed cup after cup of thick black coffee. He found that it worked best when he drank his coffee cold on an empty stomach. "Sparks shoot all the way to the brain,"[30] he declared. Eventually, even that did not give Balzac the stimulation he craved, so he took to eating dry coffee grounds.

Constricted Airways

Everybody has a uvula, the flap of soft tissue that hangs down in the back of the mouth just above the throat. The uvula plays a role in speech, vibrating as people talk. People whose uvulas are particularly long are prone to snoring because during sleep the uvula comes into contact with the throat, thereby obstructing the free flow of air in and out of the body. The uvula is one of the components of the human airway that can contribute to obstructive sleep apnea.

Also contributing to sleep apnea are the tonsils, which are located in the back of the throat. Tonsils are part of the body's immune system, trapping bacteria and releasing antibodies to fight upper respiratory infections. Years ago many people had their tonsils removed as young children because they often became infected. Now, tonsillitis is less common, and many people reach adulthood with their tonsils intact.

However, tonsils may cause snoring and sleep apnea because they can obstruct the throat. Adenoids, which perform a function similar to those of the tonsils, are glands located between the nose and throat. They can also block the airway during sleep. In apnea patients, the tongue may also slide to the back of the throat, blocking the windpipe. Finally, the weight of the neck itself can press down on the airway during sleep—a factor responsible for obstructive sleep apnea in obese men and women and athletes of large girth, such as football linemen and weight lifters.

During a sleep apnea episode, a patient's breathing will slow or completely stop. Patients may have up to 60 "apneic events" per hour, meaning they actually stop breathing 60 times per hour. In between those events, they snore. During an apneic event, the muscles in the neck relax and press down on the air passage.

Kris Jenkins, a 335-pound (152kg) defensive lineman for the Carolina Panthers, was troubled by sleep apnea for several years. His sleep was so interrupted at night that he could not help but doze off during the day. After he fell asleep during a team meeting, his coaches sent him to a doctor, who diagnosed his problem. To cure his apnea, Jenkins had his tonsils and adenoids surgically removed. "I can stay up in meetings more," Jenkins said. "It does help my breathing. I get more rest when I go to sleep. When I run around, I can breathe in more oxygen and it helps."[31]

> " During a sleep apnea episode, a patient's breathing will slow or completely stop. Patients may have up to 60 "apneic events" per hour, meaning they actually stop breathing 60 times per hour. "

The Narcoleptic Dogs

In the 1970s researchers at Stanford University noticed something unusual about dogs, particularly Doberman pinschers and Labrador retrievers. While playing fetch or begging for treats or otherwise being active and happy dogs, they suddenly collapsed, falling dead asleep. It turned out they were narcoleptic.

Over the years, the Stanford researchers gathered some 80 narcoleptic dogs, ultimately finding the reason narcoleptic people slip into sudden and deep slumbers. In 1999 they discovered a common gene in the dogs' DNA that causes narcolepsy. "These dogs laid the foundation for much of our current thinking about narcolepsy,"[32] says Thomas Scammell, a sleep researcher at Harvard University Medical School in Cambridge, Massachusetts.

The gene causes the dogs, as well as narcoleptic people, to produce too little of the hormone hypocretin, which regulates sleep and other bodily functions such as feelings of pleasure, muscle tone, and energy. Hypocretin is produced in the hypothalamus.

Scientists have not yet determined why the so-called narcoleptic gene reduces the output of hypocretin or whether there is any way to artificially enhance its production. Clearly, though, they have discovered that a lack of hypocretin is common in narcolepsy patients as well as narcoleptic dogs.

In narcoleptic people, their sleep disorder is caused by a lack of the chemical hypocretin produced by a component of the brain. Many insomniacs are affected by other physiological factors, such as blood disorders that may be making their legs feel "creepy and crawly." Or the daytime light that leaks in through the window shades in the bedroom of a night shift worker may inhibit the flow of that person's melatonin, contributing to his or her circadian rhythm disorder.

Clearly, there are many things going on inside the brain and the body that may spark sleep disorders. As science discovers more about sleep and how it is affected by the body, many more truths about sleep disorders are sure to be uncovered.

What Causes Sleep Disorders?

❝I was an infantry platoon commander in the Marine Corps. I was 23 years old, a lieutenant. Often my platoon would come back from patrols exhausted. We hadn't slept for days. The others would fall asleep on the ground, but I'd be there wiggling around with my restless legs forcing me to stay awake.❞

—Barry Kowalski, in Robert H. Yoakum, *Restless Legs Syndrome: Relief and Hope for Sleepless Victims of a Hidden Epidemic.* New York: Fireside, 2006.

Kowalksi is a Los Angeles, California, attorney and restless legs syndrome patient.

....

❝We release a sleep facilitating hormone that's called melatonin, and we release that from the pineal gland in the brain. And the timing of that is very regular if we go to sleep and wake up at the same time every night. That hormone is generally released an hour or two before we go to bed at night.❞

—Charles Czeisler, in *Charlie Rose Show*, "The Anatomy of Sleep and Sleep Disorders," MSNBC, June 5, 2006.

Czeisler is chief of the division of sleep medicine at Brigham and Women's Hospital in Boston, Massachusetts.

....

* Editor's Note: While the definition of a primary source can be narrowly or broadly defined, for the purposes of Compact Research, a primary source consists of: 1) results of original research presented by an organization or researcher; 2) eyewitness accounts of events, personal experience, or work experience; 3) first-person editorials offering pundits' opinions; 4) government officials presenting political plans and/or policies; 5) representatives of organizations presenting testimony or policy.

66 Smack in the middle of your brain is something called the pineal gland. It releases melatonin, the hormone that readies the mind and body for sleep in response to lower light levels. 99

—Mehmet C. Oz, "How to Sleep Better," *Esquire*, April 2008.

Oz is an author and professor of surgery at Columbia University Hospital in New York City.

66 Women with PMS have higher body temperatures throughout the night, and so do women who take birth control pills, which may be why birth control pills interfere with deep sleep. 99

—Gayle Greene, *Insomniac*. Berkeley and Los Angeles: University of California Press, 2008.

Greene, a professor of literature at Scripps College in Claremont, California, is an insomnia patient and author of the book *Insomniac*.

66 Coffee sets the blood in motion and stimulates the muscles; it accelerates the digestive process, chases away sleep, and gives us the capacity to engage a little longer in the exercise of our intellects. 99

—Honoré de Balzac, in Bennett Alan Weinberg and Bonnie K. Bealer, *The World of Caffeine*. New York: Routledge, 2002.

Caffeine addict Balzac was a French novelist who wrote in the nineteenth century.

❝I've got so much to do. I've got to have the caffeine.❞

—Linleigh Hawk, in Nancy Shute, "Over the Limit? Americans Young and Old Crave High-Octane Fuel, and Doctors Are Jittery," *U.S. News & World Report*, April 23, 2007. http://health.usnews.com.

Hawk is a high school senior in Potomac, Maryland, who admits to getting less than five hours of sleep a night.

❝Snoring is caused by a few things, but the biggest culprit is a vibration of very relaxed tissues in the throat, which rattle against narrow breathing passages. Symptoms are worse when you are overweight, have a short neck or still have your tonsils.❞

—Sanjay Gupta, "The Snore Wars," *Time*, September 1, 2008.

Gupta is a neurosurgeon who practices in Atlanta, Georgia, as well as a commentator and columnist on medical issues.

❝If you snore and you're overweight, you very likely have sleep apnea. And it's not the kind of snoring that's rhythmical sawing snoring, it's the kind that starts and stops—that kind of thing. Well, that's the airway opening up after it closes. We're talking about asphyxiation.❞

—Robert Basner, in *Charlie Rose Show*, "The Anatomy of Sleep and Sleep Disorders," MSNBC, June 5, 2006.

Basner is director of the Columbia University Sleep Disorder Center in New York City.

Facts and Illustrations

What Causes Sleep Disorders?

- A British study found that adolescents may have trouble falling asleep because their bodies do not start releasing **melatonin** until about 1 A.M.; in adults, melatonin is secreted around 10 P.M.

- About **25 percent** of middle-aged men and **9 percent** of middle-aged women in America suffer from sleep apnea to the degree that their throats close completely during sleep.

- Researchers in Great Britain found that **70 percent** of restless legs syndrome patients have at least one parent who also suffers from RLS, indicating that the disorder is often passed down from generation to generation.

- According to a California study, **85 percent** of snorers register 38 on the decibel scale, which is equivalent to the noise made by light highway traffic.

- About **10 percent** of the American population may suffer from some degree of restless legs syndrome, although only about **3 percent** require treatment.

- Patients of obstructive sleep apnea may have up to 60 "apneic events" per hour, meaning they **stop breathing** once every minute.

- A British study found that **45 percent** of elementary school children have trouble falling asleep; common reasons cited by the children included illnesses, anxieties over bullying at school, and other causes of stress.

- A study by researchers in Philadelphia focusing on children between the ages of 8 and 12 found that **obese children** are more susceptible to insomnia, sleep apnea, and daytime drowsiness than children who are of healthy weight.

- Nicotine, like caffeine, is a stimulant: A Maryland study of 40 smokers and 40 nonsmokers found that nearly **25 percent** of the smokers suffered from insomnia and other sleep disorders, while only **5 percent** of the nonsmokers in the study had trouble sleeping.

The Pineal Gland

The pineal gland, found deep inside the human brain, is no more than the size of a pea but plays a major role in how people sleep. The gland secretes the hormone melatonin, which induces people to fall asleep. Overnight, the pineal gland continues to release melatonin throughout slumber; as dawn approaches the production of melatonin slows, causing people to wake up.

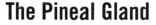

Pineal Gland

- A Wisconsin study concluded that people who drink alcoholic beverages shortly before bedtime have a **25 percent** greater risk than nondrinkers of developing sleep apnea; researchers theorized that alcohol has a constricting effect on the body's air passages.

The Importance of Circadian Rhythms

Shift workers and long-distance travelers who suffer from jet lag have trouble sleeping because their circadian rhythms are telling them it is daytime, and therefore time to wake up at a time when they would rather be sleeping. The body's circadian rhythms are controlled by the suprachiasmatic nucleus, or SCN, a cluster of cells found in a part of the brain known as the hypothalamus.

Cerebral Cortex

Suprachiasmatic Nucleus

Hypothalamus

Source: Harvard Medical School, "Under the Brain's Control," http://healthysleep.med.harvard.edu.

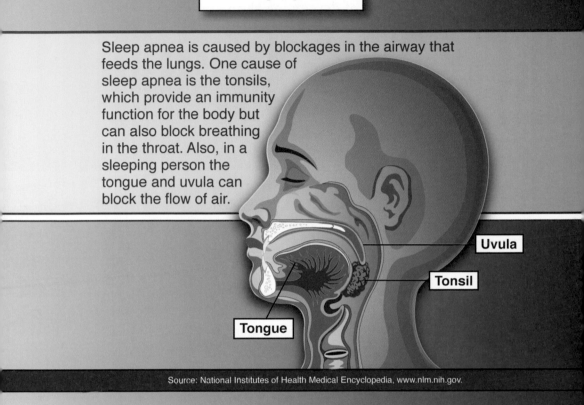

Sleep Apnea

Sleep apnea is caused by blockages in the airway that feeds the lungs. One cause of sleep apnea is the tonsils, which provide an immunity function for the body but can also block breathing in the throat. Also, in a sleeping person the tongue and uvula can block the flow of air.

Uvula

Tonsil

Tongue

Source: National Institutes of Health Medical Encyclopedia, www.nlm.nih.gov.

- About **50 percent** of middle-aged men who suffer from high blood pressure also suffer from sleep apnea.

- Between 2004 and 2007, the number of **18- to 24-year-olds** who drink at least one cup of coffee a day nearly doubled, from 16 percent to **31 percent**.

- In addition to **dogs** and humans, another species known to carry the **narcoleptic gene** is the **zebrafish**; scientists can tell the fish go narcoleptic when their tales droop.

How Do Sleep Disorders Affect People?

“**We have in our society this idea that you can just get by without sleep or manipulate when you sleep without any consequences. What we're finding is that's just not true.**”

—Lawrence Epstein, medical director of the Sleep Health Centers in Boston, Massachusetts.

In this age of 24-hour cable television, the widespread availability of the Internet, cell phones in every pocket, MP3 players plugged in to every ear, and numerous other reasons to stay up late, is it any wonder most young people simply do not get enough sleep? A 2007 study by Case Western Reserve University in Cleveland, Ohio, found that 1 in 5 middle school and high school students receive less than 6 hours of sleep a night. Optimally, doctors recommend adolescents sleep 9 hours a night.

Sleep-deprived teens often suffer from learning, health, behavioral, and mood problems. They also tend to fall asleep in class. "I've learned never to dim the lights, even to show a video," says Lauren Boyle, a history teacher at Waltham High School in Massachusetts. "If I do, there are days when a third of the class falls asleep."[33]

According to a study by the National Sleep Foundation, 28 percent of high school students admit to falling asleep in class at least once a week. "And that's the tip of the iceberg because you know they aren't alert before they fall asleep," says Amy Wolfson, an associate professor of psychology at College of the Holy Cross in Worcester, Massachusetts. "That is very alarming to me."[34]

Missing out on what the teacher says is only one of the adverse effects of poor sleep. Teens who get inadequate sleep also say they are too tired to exercise. Also, since insomnia tends to trigger a desire to eat, many teens who do not sleep well snack a lot on junk food, which could lead to obesity. "Youngsters need to be taught a healthy lifestyle includes healthy sleep as well as healthy food," says Chris Idzikowski, director of the Edinburgh Sleep Center in Scotland. "The message is simple: switch off the gadgets and get more sleep."[35]

Physical Ailments

Lack of sleep can lead to a variety of physical ailments. People who do not get enough sleep have weaker immune systems, so they tend to get more colds and flu than others.

In laboratory experiments, rats that were denied sleep over a period of three weeks died. When scientists performed autopsies on the rats, they found that the animals died from minor bacterial infections that their immune systems should have been able to fight off. Instead, the lack of sleep weakened the immune systems of the rats, contributing to their deaths. "The immune system doesn't work well if we don't sleep,"[36] says David P. White, professor of sleep medicine at Brigham and Women's Hospital in Boston.

At the University of Chicago, scientists restricted student volunteers to four hours of sleep over the course of six nights. On the seventh day, the students were administered flu vaccines. The vaccines should have prompted the students' bodies to manufacture abundant quantities of antibodies to guard them against the influenza infections, but that did not happen. Blood tests showed the vaccines in the sleep-deprived students were only half as effective as they should have been.

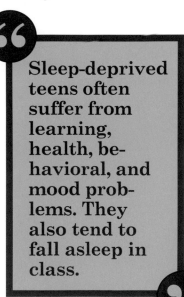

Sleep-deprived teens often suffer from learning, health, behavioral, and mood problems. They also tend to fall asleep in class.

Moreover, the heart rates and blood pressures of the sleep-deprived students were higher than normal—such factors, if continued over a long period of time, can lead to heart disease and stroke. Says Charles Czeisler of Brigham and Women's Hospital, "[When] restricted to four hours [of sleep] a night, within a couple of weeks, you could make an 18-year-old look like a 60-year-old."[37]

Mental Illnesses

Many people who are clinically depressed suffer from hypersomnia—they want to sleep all day and all night and cannot make themselves get out of bed. Other depressed and anxious people suffer from insomnia—they let their troubles dominate their lives and interrupt their sleep. Recent research indicates that while depression and other mental illnesses may cause some sleep disorders, it is possible that sleep disorders may also cause mental illnesses. "It could very well be that the increases we're seeing in some of these disorders are a direct reflection of the increasing loss of sleep in the general population,"[38] says Robert Stickgold, associate professor of psychiatry at Harvard University Medical School.

> **Sleep-deprived people do less work than others, which can be a drain on their employers.**

Stickgold says his research has also found that young children who are afflicted with sleep apnea are five times more likely than other children to also suffer from attention deficit/hyperactivity disorder, or ADHD, in which children are inattentive, impulsive, and hyperactive. Children with ADHD are often unable to function in normal social environments; they have trouble making and keeping friends, and many do poorly in school.

Episodes of mania and depression in bipolar patients may also be triggered by a lack of sleep. Bipolar patients suffer from long periods of depression interrupted by brief and erratic periods of euphoria and irritability, which reflect the manic phases of the disease. "This isn't just a small corner of the depression population," says Stickgold. "This is a lot of people that might never have been diagnosed with depression if they were able to get a good night's sleep."[39]

Women Suffer More

Women's health is affected by lack of sleep more than men's, according to a study by the University of Warwick in England. The study found that female insomniacs sustain higher degrees of high blood pressure and are more prone to heart disease than men.

University researchers studied nearly 6,600 men and women who sleep less than five hours a night. According to the study, the sleep-deprived women suffered from high blood pressure at a rate twice that of the men.

Pregnant women are often susceptible to sleep apnea because of the weight they gain during their pregnancies. A 2007 study found that pregnant women who suffer from sleep apnea are very prone to developing diabetes and high blood pressure. High blood pressure during pregnancy can lead to the conditions known as preeclampsia and eclampsia. Among the complications of preeclampsia are swelling of the feet, legs, and hands; eclampsia occurs when preeclampsia goes untreated and can lead to coma and death of the mother and her child.

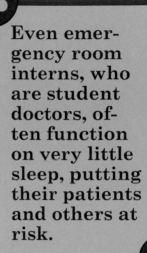

> Even emergency room interns, who are student doctors, often function on very little sleep, putting their patients and others at risk.

Moreover, sleep apnea does more than affect the mother's health—it also restricts oxygen to the fetus. Cutting off oxygen to a fetus can have devastating effects that could result in birth defects and developmental disabilities that can last the baby's lifetime. "When a mother's oxygen level drops at night, it may also affect the oxygen level of the fetus, and we don't know what the long term effects are,"[40] says Hatim Youssef, a sleep researcher at the University of Medicine and Dentistry of New Jersey.

Costs in the Workplace

When people do not get a good night's sleep, they often have trouble concentrating the next day. That means their productivity at work drops off. At Harvard University, scientists found that as many as a third of study participants who stayed awake all night had levels of concentration that were two-thirds shorter than participants who slept well.

This means that sleep-deprived people do less work than others, which can be a drain on their employers. And since they get sick more often than other employees, sleep-deprived people miss more work and incur higher health-care costs, most of which are typically paid by employer-sponsored health insurance plans. A 2007 study by Cornell University and other institutions found that employers spend some $3,200 more a year on the health-care costs of insomniacs than they do on their employees who sleep soundly. If those statistics are applied to the entire American workforce, the study suggested, the cost to the American economy would be a staggering $20 billion a year.

>
> **Drowsy driving occurs when people nod off while operating their motor vehicles. Obviously, with cars covering dozens of feet per second at high rates of speed, the results can be devastating and deadly.**

Overall, the study found that the cost to the economy—which includes health-care costs as well as lost productivity, mishaps at home, and on-the-job and car accidents—totals between $30 billion and $35 billion a year. "Our study suggests that it costs far less to treat insomnia than to ignore it," says medical statistician Ronald J. Ozminkowski, lead author of the study. "Untreated insomnia affects individuals' health, quality of life, and job performance—and increases their use of health care services substantially."[41]

Night Shift Workers

Night shift workers are prone to developing circadian rhythm disorders. Some 15 million Americans are employed in night shift jobs. The Evergreen Safety Council, which examines workplace safety issues in the Pacific Northwest, reported that as many as 20 percent of night shift workers admit to falling asleep on the job. If those employees work with heavy machinery, they may be putting themselves and others in danger.

Even emergency room interns, who are student doctors, often function on very little sleep, putting their patients and others at risk. As part of their training, new doctors are often required to work long shifts in hospital emergency rooms. Over the years, many state governments have imposed limits on the number of consecutive hours doctors may work in emergency rooms, and in 2003 the Accreditation Council for Graduate

Medical Education limited first-year interns to no more than 30 consecutive hours on duty and no more than a total of 80 hours a week. (Although the student doctors are required to be on duty for 30-hour shifts, hospitals typically permit them to take naps during slow periods.)

Nevertheless, financially burdened hospitals often ask new doctors to work longer hours. A 2006 Harvard University Medical School study found that 84 percent of nearly 1,300 first-year interns had violated the rules and worked longer shifts. The study also reported frequent mishaps occurring when the doctors worked overtime—some 1,500 doctors said they exposed themselves to contaminated bodily fluids through mishaps involving needles, scalpels, and other sharp objects.

Drowsy Driving

Drowsy driving occurs when people nod off while operating their motor vehicles. Obviously, with cars covering dozens of feet per second at high rates of speed, the results can be devastating and deadly. Indeed, some 1,500 deaths and 76,000 injuries a year are attributable to drowsy driving. Experts believe drowsy driving is just as dangerous as driving under the influence of alcohol and drugs and suggest that driving in a fatigued state is similar to driving with a blood-alcohol level of 0.10, which in all states is regarded as legally intoxicated.

According to the National Sleep Foundation, 51 percent of drivers feel sleepy at times when they are driving, while 32 percent of drivers have admitted to falling asleep behind the wheel. In 2008 one victim of drowsy driving was actor Morgan Freeman, who may have fallen asleep while driving late one night near his home in Charleston, Mississippi. Freeman's car left the highway and flipped end over end before coming to rest upright in a ditch. Freeman sustained nerve damage to an arm that took surgeons more than 4 hours to repair. Said Bill Rogers, a retired police officer who witnessed the accident and helped pull the actor from the wreck, "Mr. Freeman thought he may have gone to sleep but he wasn't sure. He didn't know what happened. The car was bent on the front as well as the rear—I mean severely. It was so bad I couldn't tell what it was."[42]

Maggie's Law

Drowsy driving incidents have led New Jersey to adopt Maggie's Law, which was named for Maggie McDonnell, a 20-year-old New Jersey college student who was killed by a drowsy driver. Maggie's Law gave police the power to charge drowsy drivers with vehicular homicide, a serious charge that carries a prison term of up to 10 years if the driver is convicted. By 2008 New Jersey was the lone state to adopt such a law, but similar laws were under consideration in Iowa, Illinois, Kentucky, Massachusetts, Michigan, New York, Oregon, and Tennessee.

Carole McDonnell recalls the accident that took the life of her daughter. "He hadn't slept for 30 hours," McDonnell says of the driver whose vehicle struck Maggie's car. "He knew he was too tired to drive. He had a choice. He chose to take a risk. He could have pulled over at that point. He chose not to. Finally, he crossed three lanes of highway and hit Maggie and killed her."[43]

Tom Callaghy, a college professor from Pennsylvania, also lost his wife to a drowsy driver. In this case, the driver was Callaghy. In 2001 Callaghy and his wife, Jane, were driving through Virginia, returning from a competition with their show dogs. Driving home late at night, Callaghy felt himself nodding off. Jane Callaghy was already asleep in the seat next to her husband. Callaghy leaned over to wake her up so she could drive, but for a moment he fell asleep. The couple's van left the road, plummeted into a gulley, and slammed into a tree. Callaghy was unhurt, but his wife was killed. He recalls:

> Janey's arm was lying on the ground in front of me. I could just barely reach it. And there was no sound from her. I couldn't tell whether she was breathing. So I reached out to check her pulse. And I didn't find any pulse. . . . We've all gotten drowsy while driving as I had, and you get through it. It's that belief that you are going to get through it again that kills.[44]

When students go without enough sleep, they may nod off in class and are likely to miss something important said by the teacher. When employees go without enough sleep, they do not perform at their best the next day. That costs their employers through lost production and increased health-care costs. When an emergency room intern is forced to work too long without sleep, he or she may make a mistake that could have a potentially devastating impact on the patient. And when a driver does not get enough sleep, the results can often be tragic—as Tom Callaghy and the family of Maggie McDonnell know all too well.

How Do Sleep Disorders Affect People?

66 There have been several studies assessing the effect of sleep deprivation. . . . In these studies, successive days of restricting sleep duration led to a significant tendency to doze off in quiet settings. This might manifest as falling asleep in class. 99

—Richard P. Millman, "Excessive Sleepiness in Adolescents and Young Adults: Causes, Consequences, and Treatment Strategies," *Pediatrics*, June 6, 2005.

A pediatrician, Millman is a member of the Working Group on Sleepiness in Adolescents for the American Academy of Pediatrics.

66 What we are seeing is the emergence of 'junk sleep'— that is, sleep that is of neither the length nor quality that it should be in order to feed the brain with the rest it needs. 99

—Chris Idzikowski, in BBC, "Junk Sleep Damaging Teen Health," August 27, 2007. http://news.bbc.co.uk.

Idzikowski, director of the Edinburgh Sleep Center in Scotland, conducted a survey of 1,000 teenagers on their sleep habits.

* Editor's Note: While the definition of a primary source can be narrowly or broadly defined, for the purposes of Compact Research, a primary source consists of: 1) results of original research presented by an organization or researcher; 2) eyewitness accounts of events, personal experience, or work experience; 3) first-person editorials offering pundits' opinions; 4) government officials presenting political plans and/or policies; 5) representatives of organizations presenting testimony or policy.

❝Lack of sleep disrupts every physiologic function of the body. We have nothing in our body that allows us to adapt to this behavior.❞

—Eve Van Cauter, in Rob Stein, "Too Little Sleep Taking a Toll on America's Health," *Buffalo News*, October 30, 2005.

Van Cauter is a sleep researcher at the University of Chicago.

❝There are Chicken Little people running around saying that the sky is falling because people are not sleeping enough. But everyone knows people are getting healthier. Life expectancy has been increasing, and people are healthier today than they were generations ago.❞

—Daniel F. Kripke, in Rob Stein, "Too Little Sleep Taking a Toll on America's Health," *Buffalo News*, October 30, 2005.

Kripke is a professor of psychiatry at the University of California at San Diego.

❝We often automatically retreat to bed when we have a cold or sore throat, instinctively perceiving that sleep helps us heal. Growing evidence suggests this is not mere wishful thinking but scientific fact.❞

—National Sleep Foundation, *Sleep-Wake Cycle: Its Physiology and Impact on Health*, 2006.

The National Sleep Foundation supports research into sleep disorders and provides information to the public as well as training for health-care providers on sleep disorders.

❝I don't want to deal with things because I'm afraid of not being able to do it rationally or logically. I know myself, and I don't want to react badly or do something I might regret.❞

—Margaret Chau, in Erin Allady, "The Science of Sleep Deprivation," *San Francisco Chronicle*, October 23, 2007.

Chau, who lives in Millbrae, California, and suffers from chronic insomnia due to back pain, describes how she feels after a sleepless night.

....

❝One of the functions of sleep is to reset and replenish the emotional integrity of our brain circuits so we can approach the day's emotional challenges in appropriate ways. If you don't get a good night's sleep, you'll be making irrational choices.❞

—Matthew Walker, in Erin Allady, "The Science of Sleep Deprivation," *San Francisco Chronicle*, October 23, 2007.

Walker is director of the University of California at Berkeley Sleep and Neuroimaging Laboratory.

....

❝When we are sleep deprived, we think and move more slowly, make more mistakes, and have difficulty remembering things. This leads to lower productivity and can cause work related accidents.❞

—Tom Odegaard, "Shift Workers and Sleep," *Safety and Health Solutions*, February 2007.

Odegaard is executive director of the Evergreen Safety Council of Seattle, Washington.

....

66 **When you're behind the wheel of a car, it's a 3,000-pound killing machine, and if you're not fully alert, you can either kill someone else, kill yourself or do jail time.** 99

—Darrel Drobnich, in CBS News, "Waking Up to Drowsy-Driving Danger," October 20, 2004. www.cbsnews.com.

Drobnich is chief program officer of the National Sleep Foundation.

66 **Over-the-road trucking has long been thought to be an area of great concern. Since drowsy drivers are every bit as common as drunk drivers, the trucker who is hauling a huge rig and is affected by sleep apnea is a major risk.** 99

—Ron Baake, in *Small Business Times*, "Company to Monitor Truckers' Sleep Disorders," October 3, 2008. www.biztimes.com.

Baake is chief executive officer of the Sleep Wellness Institute of West Allis, Wisconsin, which was retained to diagnose and treat sleep apnea in drivers employed by a Wisconsin trucking company.

How Do Sleep Disorders Affect People?

- A California study found that the interruption in breathing during sleep apnea events can cause brain damage; in 43 sleep apnea patients, parts of the brain known as mammillary bodies, which relay thoughts to other parts of the brain, were **20 percent** smaller than in non-apnea patients.

- In an Illinois study, after just two nights, men restricted to four hours of sleep per night had an **18 percent** decrease in leptin, the hormone that signals an end to hunger after eating, and a **28 percent** increase in ghrelin, the hormone that triggers hunger.

- According to *Newsweek*, the average twelfth grader has **four major electronic devices**, such as televisions or stereos, in his or her bedroom.

- A Texas study found that adolescents who suffer from insomnia are **2.3 times** more likely than other young people to develop symptoms of depression in early adulthood.

- A report by the U.S. Surgeon General concluded that sleep disorders add **$15 billion** to national health-care costs and trim worker productivity by **$50 billion** a year.

- National studies show that sleep apnea patients are 4 times more likely than others to suffer a **stroke** and 3 times more likely than others to suffer **heart disease**.

- A national study found that **28 percent** of high school students admit to falling asleep in class at least once a week; **22 percent** say they fall asleep doing their homework.

Sleep Disorders Affect Job Performance

Nearly 30 percent of American workers admit to falling asleep on the job from time to time because they have not gotten enough sleep the night before. A small percentage admit to being late for work because of sleepless nights, leaving early because they didn't feel like working, and even staying home and missing work because of insomnia or other sleep disorders.

Legend:
- 1 or more
- None
- Don't know/Refused

Number of Times . . . Due to Sleepiness or Sleep Problems in Past Month

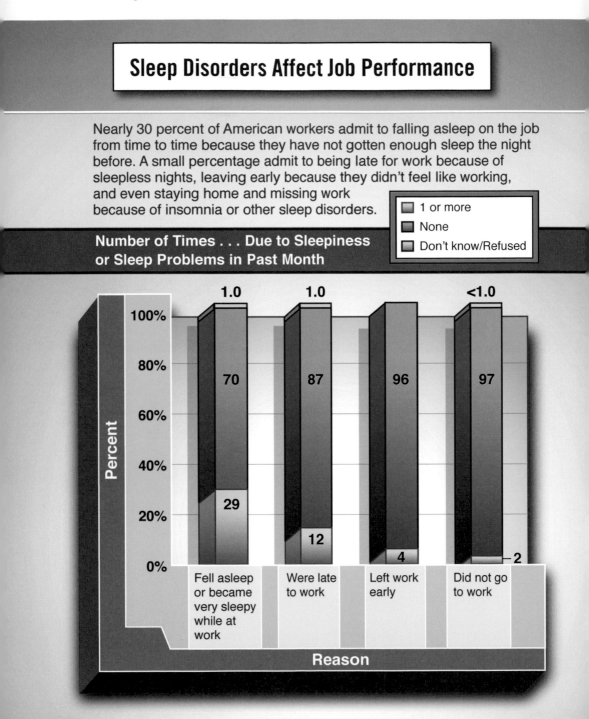

Reason	1 or more	None
Fell asleep or became very sleepy while at work	29	70 (1.0)
Were late to work	12	87 (1.0)
Left work early	4	96 (<1.0)
Did not go to work	2	97

Source: National Sleep Foundation, *2008 Sleep in America Poll*, 2008. www.sleepfoundation.org.

Most People Do Not Get Recommended Amount of Sleep

Even as young children, people do not get the amount of sleep recommended by experts. The deficit really grows in adolescence: Teenagers are believed to have too many distractions—friends, television, the Internet, and schoolwork—and not enough time for sleep. Indeed, most teenagers get less than 8 hours of sleep a night on school nights although sleep experts insist that young people need 9 hours or more of sleep.

Age	Natural Bedtime	Recommended Hours of Sleep	Actual Hours of Sleep
0–1 years	7–8 PM	14–15 hours	12.8 hours
1–2 years	7–8 PM	12–14 hours	11.8 hours
3–6 years	7–8 PM	11–13 hours	10.3 hours
7–11 years	8–9 PM	10–11 hours	9.4 hours
12–17 years	10:30–11:30 PM	8.5–9.5 hours	7.6 weekdays 8.9 weekends
18–54 years	10 PM–12 AM	7–8.5 hours	6.8 weekdays 7.4 weekends
55–84 years	8–10 PM	7–8.5 hours	6.9 weekdays 7.5 weekends

Source: Lawrence Epstein and Steven Mardon, "Homeroom Zombies," *Newsweek*, September 17, 2007, p. 64.

- Driving by drowsy drivers causes more than **1,500 deaths** and **76,000 injuries** a year, according to statistics compiled by the federal government.

- Some **32 million** people have admitted to falling asleep while driving motor vehicles.

- According to a Rhode Island study, **1 in 5** students between 11 and 17 get the recommended 9 hours of sleep a night, and **50 percent** get less than 8 hours on school nights.

Driving While Tired Is Dangerous

Nearly a third of all drivers admit to falling asleep at the wheel at least once a month, with some drivers admitting that they doze off while driving 3 times a week or more. Meanwhile, 2 percent of drivers admit that they have caused accidents because they drove while drowsy. Experts believe drowsy driving is just as dangerous as driving under the influence of alcohol or drugs and suggest that driving fatigued is similar to driving with a blood-alcohol level of .10, which in all states is legally intoxicated.

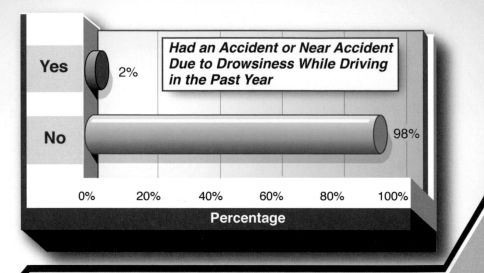

Had an Accident or Near Accident Due to Drowsiness While Driving in the Past Year

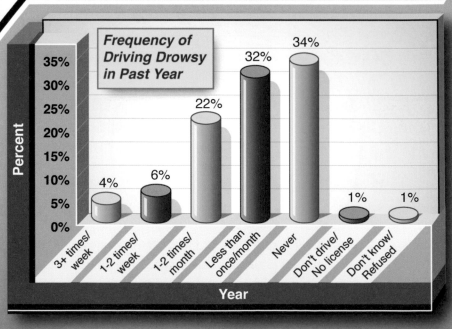

Frequency of Driving Drowsy in Past Year

Source: National Sleep Foundation, *2008 Sleep in America Poll*, 2008. www.sleepfoundation.org.

Tired Student Doctors Cause Injuries

Medical interns, who are student doctors, often have to work shifts in emergency rooms for 30 hours or more, a situation that has been cited as a major factor in injuries sustained by the interns, hospital employees, and patients. Frequently, the injuries are caused by mishaps involving scalpels and needles. Sleep researchers questioned emergency room interns involved in 448 such mishaps to find out the causes, and in a majority of the cases the interns said they had either a lapse in concentration or were suffering fatigue. Both are conditions that can be caused by lack of sleep.

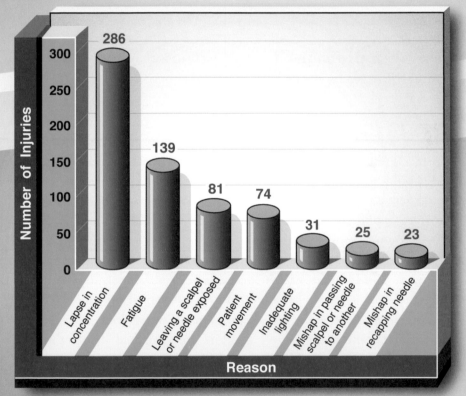

Note: The statistics add up to more than 448 because in some cases, two or more factors were cited as causing the mishap.

Source: Najib T. Ayas et al., "Extended Work Duration and the Risk of Self-Reported Percutaneous Injuries in Interns," *Journal of the American Medical Association*, September 6, 2006, p. 1,058.

- Staying awake for 24 hours has the same effect on **coordination and reaction time** as drinking alcoholic beverages to the point of intoxication, according to Harvard University sleep researchers.

Can People
Overcome Sleep
Disorders?

" Most sleep problems are self-inflicted by sleepers not knowing how to sleep. "

—Peter Bils, an executive with the American mattress company Select Comfort.

Sleep experts advocate that if a person cannot fall asleep within 15 to 20 minutes, or wakes up and cannot fall back to sleep, he or she should not remain in bed, tossing and turning. Rather, the person should get out of bed and find something relaxing to do, such as reading a book or taking a warm bath. "If you're still awake after 15 minutes, get up and do something quiet, like reading a book," says Mehmet C. Oz, an author and professor of surgery at Columbia University Hospital in New York City. "No Internet, no TV, no exercise. You have to let your body and mind slow down to be able to slip into sleep. If you just lie there thinking about how you're not sleeping, you'll never sleep."[45]

A big mistake many people make is going to bed before they are sleepy. In fact, one technique recommended for insomniacs is known as sleep restriction therapy, which works by limiting the hours the person spends in bed. If an insomniac has a difficult night and sleeps for just 4 hours while tossing and turning for another 4 hours, the patient would be instructed to spend just 4 hours in bed the next night—the patient would stay up until 2 A.M., then set his or her alarm clock for 6 A.M.

Under sleep restriction therapy, the time the patient spends in bed should become more restful—if the therapy works, the patient will sleep for nearly the entire 4 hours. The next night, the patient may want to try spending an additional 15 minutes in bed. Eventually, the patient may be able to extend his or her restful hours in bed to a full 7 or 8 hours. Says

Mark Mahowald, director of the Minnesota Regional Sleep Disorders Center, "The more you stay in bed and try to force yourself to sleep, the more you won't be able to. This gets reinforced every single night."[46]

Over-the-Counter Remedies

For insomniacs who need the help of sleeping pills, drug therapy has advanced well beyond the days when doctors prescribed barbiturates to help their patients sleep. There are many nonprescription sleeping aids available in drug stores. Some are similar to allergy medications, which work by blocking histamines. Histamines are chemicals released by the body's immune system. Most people will experience a histamine reaction to an insect bite—the histamines are what cause the bite to swell into a bump, which agitates nerves and makes the bump itch. In hay fever sufferers, the histamines are what cause runny noses and watery eyes. To make these symptoms go away, people can take an antihistamine, such as Benadryl, which neutralizes the histamines.

Histamines also tend to promote wakefulness; therefore, in many people, antihistamines may cause drowsiness. Many insomniacs who turn to drugs will first try a nonprescription antihistamine, such as Benadryl or pills marketed specifically as sleep aids, such as Nytol or Sominex. Some nonprescription painkillers have also been manufactured containing antihistamines so that people who suffer from minor pain can fall asleep. The manufacturers of those products and similar antihistamine medications market them as treatments for occasional sleeplessness—chronic insomniacs often find they need stronger medicine.

> " A big mistake many people make is going to bed before they are sleepy. "

Another nonprescription sleep medicine is melatonin, the hormone that is secreted when the body's circadian clock signals bedtime. Melatonin can be manufactured artificially and taken in pill form. Studies have shown mixed results on its effectiveness. Some people whose sleep is interrupted by jet lag have found melatonin helps them fall asleep when darkness falls in their new time zones, while others have found melatonin supplements provide minimal or no assistance in helping them fall asleep. Says *Insomniac* author Gayle Greene,

"Most researchers acknowledge that it helps with jet lag and that it may help insomnia when the problem is associated with a circadian problem or with difficulty initiating sleep; but evidence for its effectiveness with sleep maintenance insomnia is mixed."[47]

Prescription Drugs

For insomniacs who need something stronger than a melatonin supplement or an antihistamine, a class of prescription medications known as benzodiazepines has been available for several years. Psychiatrists have prescribed benzodiazepines such as Valium to treat anxiety in their patients. These drugs enhance the release of the neurotransmitter gamma-aminobutyric acid, or GABA, which slows down brain activity. By enhancing the flow of GABA in brain cells, benzodiazepines can have a calming effect on anxieties. As a side effect, benzodiazepines can cause drowsiness. These drugs have addictive qualities, which is why doctors usually write prescriptions for the drugs in small doses.

Recently, a new class of pills known as Z drugs has emerged, including Lunesta and Ambien. These drugs work by slowing down the electrical activity in the brain. (They are known as "Z drugs" because of the *z*'s in their generic names—Ambien's generic name is zolpidem while Lunesta's is eszopiclone.) Like benzodiazepines, the Z drugs enhance the release of GABA. They are considered to have a much more powerful impact on GABA than the benzodiazepines and are regarded as less habit-forming. Also, unlike benzodiazepines, they do not cause next-day grogginess. Other people with sleep disorders have also turned to prescription medication. Narcoleptics often take stimulants such as Ritalin to help them stay awake during the day. Stimulants enhance the release of the neurotransmitter dopamine, giving the brain a jolt of energy. Restless legs syndrome patients often find that the drug ropinirole, which is marketed most familiarly as Requip, provides relief from

Reggie White, the former NFL star whose sleep apnea contributed to his fatal heart attack, had a CPAP mask, but he often did not wear it to bed because he found it uncomfortable.

their symptoms. Ropinirole also enhances dopamine, which can calm body movements. In the past, ropinirole has been prescribed as a treatment for Parkinson's disease; a symptom of Parkinson's is muscle tremors.

Help for Sleep Apnea Patients

At one time the only relief for a sleep apnea patient was a tracheotomy, in which a tube is surgically implanted in the throat. In recent years, researchers have developed the continuous positive airway pressure (CPAP) mask, which uses an electric pump to blow air into the patient's mouth during sleep. The increased air pressure in the mouth helps keep the throat open during sleep. Indeed, the CPAP is regarded as the first line of defense against obstructive sleep apnea. Reggie White, the former NFL star whose sleep apnea contributed to his fatal heart attack, had a CPAP mask, but he often did not wear it to bed because he found it uncomfortable.

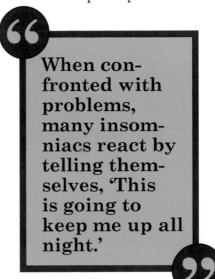

When confronted with problems, many insomniacs react by telling themselves, 'This is going to keep me up all night.'

Still, many sleep apnea patients vouch for its effectiveness. *Time* magazine correspondent Andrew Sullivan suffered from sleep apnea for many years. Finally, he spent a night in a sleep clinic, where his symptoms were monitored and he learned how to use a CPAP mask. Wrote Sullivan:

> In the morning I had a truly unexpected sensation. The nurse woke me at 5:45 A.M., a time of day I hadn't really experienced since high school. And I felt fine. More than fine, actually. I felt like a 10-year-old after a cappuccino. Since I normally take a couple of hours after I wake up (around 10 A.M.) to arrive at even moderate alertness, I was stunned. What had happened? A week later, I got the results from the sleep clinic. Without the CPAP, I had stopped breathing an average 38 times an hour. I had got absolutely no stage 4 sleep, the kind that really refreshes your mind and body. With the CPAP machine, I breathed normally, and 17 percent of my sleep was stage 4. No wonder I felt better.[48]

Also available to sleep apnea patients is a dental appliance known as the mandibular advancement device, which shifts the jaw slightly, opening the airway; and a minor surgical procedure, uvulopalatopharyngoplasty, in which the patient's uvula is trimmed.

Treatment for Parasomniacs

The treatment for sleepwalking can be very simple—many doctors advise their patients to lock their bedroom doors before turning off the lights. That way, at least, the somnambulists will stay in their rooms during their sleepwalking episodes.

Somnambulists are also known to walk in their sleep at the same time each night. Therefore, physicians recommend waking up the sleepwalker 15 minutes before the anticipated episode. After a few weeks on such a schedule, the sleepwalking episodes usually disappear.

Hypnotherapy is regarded as an effective treatment for sleepwalking as well as for sleep terrors and nightmare disorders. When practiced by a psychiatrist or psychologist, hypnotherapy can plant a suggestive notion in the memory of a patient that can be employed to alter physical behavior. Many people find hypnotherapy is effective in helping them quit smoking—the notion planted by the therapists leads them to believe smoking is a repugnant habit.

The same techniques have been employed to convince people not to be frightened of their dreams, a reaction that often acts as the trigger for sleepwalking and other parasomnia disorders. Said the authors of a 2007 study on the effectiveness of hypnotherapy in 36 parasomniac patients: "The results indicate that one month after hypnotherapy, close to half of the study patients showed either no parasomnia events or at least rated themselves as much improved. It seems likely that this short-term effect is a direct consequence of the hypnotherapy."[49]

Cognitive Behavioral Therapy

Psychotherapy may provide help for other patients who suffer from sleep disorders. Psychotherapists who work with insomniacs often employ the techniques of cognitive behavioral therapy, or CBT.

CBT has been used for decades by mental health professionals to treat people who suffer from phobias and other irrational fears. Such patients often fear social situations or specific activities, such as flying or riding in elevators. Under the therapy, phobic patients learn what troubles them and how to overcome their fears in small steps. A person who fears heights may take an elevator to the second floor on the first day of his or her therapy, the fourth floor on the second day, the ninth floor on the third day, and so on until the patient reaches the top floor of a skyscraper.

Sleep disorder patients can benefit from the same type of therapy. Under CBT, insomniacs learn what causes their sleeplessness while also learning strategies for confronting anxieties and other causes of stress and learning to deal with them in ways that do not cost them sleep. In many cases, CBT patients learn to address their problems with positive outlooks. When confronted with problems, many insomniacs react by telling themselves, "This is going to keep me up all night." By practicing cognitive behavioral therapy, patients learn to find positive responses to those stresses. Says John W. Winkelman, a sleep researcher at Brigham and Women's Hospital:

> **There are more than 1,400 sleep clinics in America, employing teams of specialists who treat insomnia as well as other sleep disorders, including narcolepsy and sleep apnea.**

> They . . . become more confident about falling asleep at the beginning of the night or at nighttime awakenings, which counteracts the anxiety about sleeplessness—the real enemy of persons with insomnia. The cognitive aspect of the therapy helps bolster this confidence. Cognitive behavioral therapy addresses the anxieties about sleeplessness and the catastrophic beliefs about what is going to happen.[50]

Sleep Clinics

Years ago people who could not sleep were left virtually on their own when it came to finding cures for their sleep disorders, or they were forced to take one of the few addictive knockout drugs known to be effective sleep aids. Although doctors and research scientists had been studying sleep for centuries, it took until 1970 for the first clinic to be established specifically to treat sleep disorders. That institution, the Stanford University Sleep Disorders Clinic in California, has gone on to treat thousands of patients.

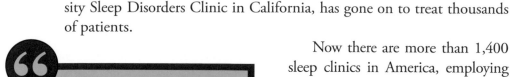

Experts agree that the best way to enjoy a good night's sleep is to practice good sleep hygiene. They urge people to use their beds only for sleeping: no TV, no video games, no cell phone chats, and no Internet use in bed, particularly late at night and shortly before bedtime.

Now there are more than 1,400 sleep clinics in America, employing teams of specialists who treat insomnia as well as other sleep disorders, including narcolepsy and sleep apnea. Typically, patients spend the night at the clinics, where physicians and nurses monitor their sleep and help diagnose their disorders. As the patient sleeps, he or she will be hooked to machines that monitor pulse rate, blood pressure, brain activity, breathing, and other bodily functions. These tests are known as polysomnograms.

During a visit to a sleep clinic, *New York Times* reporter William L. Hamilton learned he had sleep apnea. The condition had been interrupting his breathing 16 times per hour while he slept. He described the experience of sleeping at the clinic:

During the night, as I traveled between wakefulness and sleep, sending back streams of data like a space probe, the technician appeared and disappeared, adjusting my wires, and exiting my consciousness in a ring of light—the door to the corridor—like a special visitor, a goblin that only the sixth-sensed see. He monitored my voyage from a desk somewhere in the clinic, taking notes as I sped through the blackness.[51]

Hamilton was urged by his doctor to wear a CPAP mask at night. Some 75 percent of severe apnea patients agree to wear the masks after their diagnoses at sleep clinics or in their doctors' offices.

What Is Good Sleep Hygiene?

While there may be many drugs and other medical therapies available for people to help them sleep, experts agree that the best way to enjoy a good night's sleep is to practice good sleep hygiene. They urge people to use their beds only for sleeping: no TV, no video games, no cell phone chats, and no Internet use in bed, particularly late at night and shortly before bedtime. Says Jean Matheson, medical director of the Sleep Disorders Center at Beth Israel Deaconess Medical Center in Boston: "A huge amount of insomnia is induced by behaviors that can be quickly fixed. . . . People think night just happens, but the way you sleep is often reflective of your health and activities during the day: how you wake up, what the room is like, what you do when you get up, when you have coffee, your routine when you come home."[52]

According to the National Sleep Foundation, here are some examples of good sleep hygiene:

- Maintain a regular schedule of going to bed and getting up in the morning, even on weekends. Sleeping late on Saturdays and Sundays may upset the sleeper's circadian clock; on Sunday night, the person may not be sleepy at bedtime even though he or she has to get up early for school or work Monday morning.

- Establish a regular routine for bedtime, such as reading or listening to soft music shortly before lights out. A relaxing routine may help dispel the anxieties that have accumulated during the day.

- The bedroom should be sleep conducive, free of noise and other distractions such as bright lights. The mattress should be comfortable.

- Finish eating at least two or three hours before bed. A full stomach may make it hard to rest late at night; also, consuming too many fluids in the evening may cause frequent trips to the bathroom overnight. People should be particularly careful to stay away from coffee and other caffeinated drinks late at night.

- Alcoholic beverages should also be avoided near bedtime—although drinking may initially make people drowsy, alcohol causes thirst and enhances the urge to urinate, two conditions known to interrupt sleep.

Certainly, some sleep disorders are unavoidable and unconnected to sleep hygiene: the causes of narcolepsy, hypersomnia, parasomnia, and sleep apnea, among others, are beyond the control of the patients who must turn to drugs, psychotherapy, and other medical procedures to relieve their symptoms. But for the vast majority of sleep disorder patients—some 60 million insomnia-suffering Americans who lie awake at night, watching the minutes tick off their digital clocks—experts agree that many can find relief if they simply learn how to turn off their TV sets, pull down the shades, and leave their anxieties at their bedroom doors.

Can People Overcome Sleep Disorders?

"Sleep becomes more predictable. You build up a sleep drive because you cut yourself short of bed rest."

—Paul Glovinsky, in *Providence Journal*, "The Essentials," October 10, 2005.

Glovinsky, an advocate of sleep restriction therapy, is clinical director of Capital Region Sleep-Wake Disorders Center in Albany, New York.

"A little chemical help once in a while is fine. Not alcohol—it actually interferes with the normal sleep cycle. But Benadryl or one of the combination over-the-counter painkillers or sleep drugs can give you that little nudge into natural sleep."

—Mehmet C. Oz, "How to Sleep Better," *Esquire*, April 2008.

Oz is an author and professor of surgery at Columbia University Hospital in New York City.

* Editor's Note: While the definition of a primary source can be narrowly or broadly defined, for the purposes of Compact Research, a primary source consists of: 1) results of original research presented by an organization or researcher; 2) eyewitness accounts of events, personal experience, or work experience; 3) first-person editorials offering pundits' opinions; 4) government officials presenting political plans and/or policies; 5) representatives of organizations presenting testimony or policy.

❝Ambien is relatively effective in the short term, but [you've] really got to find the underlying cause. Why would people want to take a pill to sleep for the rest of their life?❞

—Daniel Salzman, in Shazia Ahmad, "Generation Zzzzzz," *New York Observer*, April 25, 2005.

Salzman is a sleep specialist at the New York Presbyterian Hospital Sleep-Wake Disorders Center in White Plains, New York.

❝There is such a huge, untapped market of insomniacs out there who aren't seeking treatment, or who are getting suboptimal treatment.❞

—David Southwell, in Gayle Greene, *Insomniac.* Berkeley and Los Angeles: University of California Press, 2008.

Southwell is an executive for Sepracor, manufacturer of the prescription sleep aid Lunesta.

❝I have been using the CPAP machine for several months now. Apart from a few minor side effects—dry, stuffy nose, minor irritation to the skin on my face, and some minor irritation to my eyes—I have done very well. It's not a noisy machine. Both my wife and I have gotten used to the gentle machine noise. I feel 100 percent better. I have much more energy.❞

—Ralph E. Dittman, "Sleep Apnea: A Wake-Up Call," *Saturday Evening Post*, May/June 2007.

Dittman is a research scientist at Baylor College of Medicine in Houston, Texas, and a sleep apnea patient.

66 After a poor night of sleep we're asking people to forget about it and go about their business as usual because if you wake up and think, 'Wow, what a terrible night of sleep, I'm going to have a lousy day,' you're setting yourself up for failure. **99**

—Charles Morin, in Jon Mooallem, "The Sleep-Industrial Complex," *New York Times Magazine*, November 18, 2007.

Morin is a psychologist at Laval University in Quebec City, Canada, and an advocate for treating insomniacs with cognitive behavioral therapy.

66 Night after night, I've watched people in our lab and our clinic undergo the commonplace and profound transformation called falling asleep. **99**

—William Dement, in Tracie White, "Stalking the Netherworld of Sleep," *Stanford Report*, July 23, 2008. http://news-service. stanford.edu.

Dement is the founder of the Stanford University Sleep Disorders Clinic in California.

66 Our sleep-wake cycle is regulated by a 'circadian clock' in our brain and the body's need to balance both sleep time and wake time. A regular waking time in the morning strengthens the circadian function and can help with sleep onset at night. That is also why it is important to keep a regular bedtime and wake-time, even on weekends when there is temptation to sleep in. **99**

—National Sleep Foundation, "Healthy Sleep Tips." www.sleepfoundation.org.

The National Sleep Foundation supports research into sleep disorders and provides information to the public as well as training for health-care providers on sleep disorders.

66 If you fall asleep with the television on, an hour or so later it's still on and wakes you up. Many people don't like falling asleep without some sound. For them, I suggest something uniform and less entertaining, such as the sound of waves or classical music. It should be on a timer, so that it turns off after you fall asleep. 99

—John W. Winkelman, in Patrick Perry, "To Sleep, Perchance to Dream," *Saturday Evening Post*, July/August 2007.

Winkelman is a sleep researcher at Brigham and Women's Hospital in Boston, Massachusetts.

66 It's the caffeine, stupid! Anyone who has trouble sleeping should avoid caffeinated drinks and chocolate. There is evidence that caffeine intensifies restless legs syndrome in children and perhaps in some adults. 99

—Robert H. Yoakum, *Restless Legs Syndrome: Relief and Hope for Sleepless Victims of a Hidden Epidemic.* New York: Fireside, 2006.

Yoakum, an author and restless legs syndrome patient, is a founder of the Restless Legs Syndrome Foundation of Rochester, Minnesota.

Facts and Illustrations

Can People Overcome Sleep Disorders?

- Nutritionists urge long-distance travelers to eat **dried cherries** during their flights: the *New York Times* reported that cherries contain large quantities of melatonin, which can help reset the circadian clocks of travelers who suffer jet leg after crossing many time zones.

- Each year, physicians write some **49 million** prescriptions for sleeping pills.

- **Fifty percent** of 11- and 12-year-olds in the city of Adelaide, Australia, play video games, watch TV, or listen to music before they fall asleep each night, according to an Australian study.

- Ambien generates some **$1.7 billion** a year in sales for its manufacturer, Sanofi-Aventis U.S., of Bridgewater, New Jersey; sales of all Z drugs total about **$2.8 billion** a year.

- There are more than **1,400** clinics in America specializing in the treatment of sleep disorders; in 1970, there was one.

- A study reported by the *New York Times* found that, on the average, **Ambien** users fell asleep just **23 minutes** faster than study participants taking a placebo.

- Canadian researchers believe a regular sleep schedule may help prevent somnambulism: According to a Montreal study, **90 percent** of

Treating Sleep Apnea with a CPAP Mask

The process known as continuous positive airway pressure, or CPAP, pumps air into the mouth of the sleep apnea patient overnight. The increased air pressure in the mouth forces open the body's air passage, preventing it from closing during sleep apnea episodes. The CPAP machine consists of a small air pump, hose, and mask that fits over the nose, or both mouth and nose, depending on the severity of the patient's sleep apnea. Physicians regard the CPAP mask as the first line of defense against sleep apnea, which can be fatal by causing the patient to stop breathing, often dozens of times an hour.

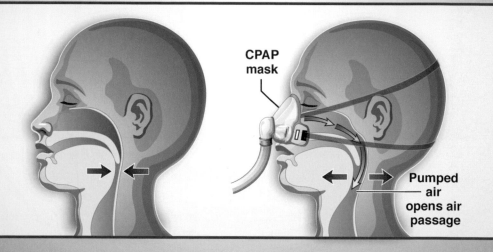

CPAP mask

Pumped air opens air passage

Source: Medical College of Wisconsin, "Treatments of Obstructive Sleep Apnea," www.mcw.edu.

patients who stayed awake for 25 hours experienced a sleepwalking episode when they were finally permitted to sleep.

- **Counting sheep** falls short of other methods for falling asleep, a British study concluded. Insomniacs who were told to fall asleep while counting sheep took longer to nod off than insomniacs who were instructed to imagine a relaxing scene.

- A Norwegian study found that over a six-month period, cognitive behavioral therapy improved the sleep duration of insomnia patients by **52 percent**; during that same period, patients who took Z drugs saw their sleep duration improve by **16 percent**.

Prescription Medications Help Most People Sleep

In a survey of more than 2,000 insomnia patients, *Consumer Reports* magazine found that most feel that taking prescription drugs is the most effective treatment that helps them fall asleep. Using sound machines—devices that simulate the sounds of ocean waves, rainfall, and other pleasant noises—is nearly as effective as sleeping pills, the magazine reported. Less effective is maintaining a consistent routine of going to bed and rising at the same time each day, and using muscle relaxation exercises, such as clenching and unclenching muscles in arms, legs, necks, and shoulders, before bedtime.

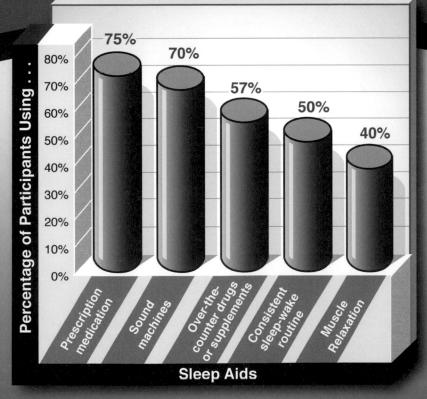

Source: *Consumer Reports*, "How Did You Sleep Last Night?" September 2008, p. 12.

- A study by German sleep researchers found that people whose bodies are oriented **north-south** during sleep have longer periods of rapid eye movement (REM) sleep than people whose bodies are oriented **east-west**; the researchers speculated that the earth's magnetism may have some effect on enhancing REM sleep.

- There is truth to the notion that a glass of **warm milk** before bed can help induce sleep; a California study found that milk contains the protein alpha-lactalbumin, which enhances the signal notifying the brain it is time to sleep.

Key People and Advocacy Groups

American Insomnia Association: Established by patients afflicted with insomnia and their physicians, the American Insomnia Association helps patients find the best treatments for their sleep disorders. The association advises members on how to use medications and other therapies to treat insomnia.

American Sleep Apnea Association: The organization helps sleep apnea patients find treatments for their afflictions, providing public information resources on medications, surgeries, and continuous positive airway pressure (CPAP) masks. The association also coordinates the activities of numerous local support groups that help sleep apnea patients find treatment.

Better Sleep Council: Sponsored by American mattress manufacturers, the Better Sleep Council helps consumers make choices about which mattresses are best suited to their needs. The council also sponsors research on the development of mattress technology.

CPAP Society: Established by users of continuous positive airway pressure (CPAP) devices, the CPAP Society provides forums for members to discuss their problems and solutions to sleep apnea. The society also provides a clearinghouse for news about sleep apnea and development of CPAP technology.

Charles Czeisler: Head of the Sleep Medicine Division at Brigham and Women's Hospital in Boston, Massachusetts, Czeisler was the first neuroscientist to determine the affect of light on the body's circadian clock. Czeisler concluded that the brain knows it is bedtime because of a lack of light entering the eyes late at night. Czeisler has devoted himself to convincing people, particularly adolescents and young children, to get more sleep.

William Dement: Known as the "Sandman," Dement established the first sleep disorders clinic at Stanford University Hospital in 1970.

Dement was a member of the team of physicians at the University of Chicago in the 1950s that discovered rapid eye movement (REM) sleep, the stage of sleep in which the eye moves rapidly under the closed eyelid while the brain is busy dreaming. That discovery launched Dement on his lifelong quest to uncover new truths about sleep.

Drowsydriving.org: Sponsored by the National Sleep Foundation, Drowsydriving.org tracks legislative efforts to enact state and federal laws that prohibit drowsy driving in America. The group also sponsors Drowsy Driving Prevention Week each November and underwrites other public information campaigns to alert the public of the dangers of drowsy driving.

Karl A. Ekbom: Born in 1907, the Swedish neurologist was the first to diagnose restless legs syndrome in 8 patients who complained of unpleasant sensations in their legs that kept them up nights. In 1945 Ekbom described the disorder as "restless legs," but the ailment was initially known as "Ekbom's disease" until doctors became more familiar with its symptoms, giving it the familiar name of "restless legs syndrome." Ekbom died in 1977.

Maggie McDonnell: The death of the 20-year-old college student in a collision caused by a drowsy driver prompted authorities in New Jersey to adopt the nation's first law enabling police to charge drowsy drivers with vehicular homicide in cases in which they cause fatal accidents. On July 2, 1997, McDonnell was heading to work at 11:30 in the morning when her car was struck by a vehicle driven by a man who later admitted he had not slept for 30 hours. Since there was no law linking his conduct with vehicular homicide, the only sentence the court could impose on the guilty driver was a suspended jail sentence and a $200 fine.

Narcolepsy Network: Established in 1986, the Narcolepsy Network helps patients understand their symptoms and seek treatment for narcolepsy. The network also helps patients understand their employment and housing rights and serves as a clearinghouse for news and developments in the treatment of the affliction.

Henri Piéron: A 1913 book by the French physician was the first to suggest that insomnia and other sleep disorders could be sparked by physiological causes, thus establishing that sleep disorders were common ailments that could be treated by doctors. Born in 1881, Piéron showed that chemicals in the body, such as neurotransmitters and hormones, affect how people sleep. Piéron died in 1964.

Restless Legs Syndrome Foundation: The Restless Legs Syndrome Foundation helps patients learn about the symptoms and therapies for the affliction. The foundation also helps patients find support groups in their hometowns, raises money for research, and provides public information on the syndrome.

Chronology

Early 1600s
William Shakespeare writes *Macbeth*, a tragedy about a king who commits murder to attain the throne; in the play, Macbeth, tortured by the anxieties of his crime, suffers from insomnia.

1735
Benjamin Franklin, a lifelong insomniac, encourages colonial Americans to get a good night's sleep when he publishes the proverb "Early to bed and early to rise, makes a man healthy, wealthy and wise" in *Poor Richard's Almanack*.

1906
Congress adopts the U.S. Pure Food and Drug Act, essentially putting an end to the patent medicine trade in America, which had produced a number of narcotic and addictive sleep aids, including laudanum, which is composed of alcohol and opium.

1950s
Experimenting on fruit flies, Princeton University biologist Colin Pittendrigh discovers the circadian clock that tells the brain when it is night and day.

1850   **1875**   **1900**   **1925**   **1950**

1879
Thomas Edison invents the incandescent lightbulb, making it possible for people to work and do other activities late into the night, thus depriving themselves of sleep.

1913
French physician Henri Piéron publishes a study suggesting sleep problems could be attributed to physiological reasons, thereby establishing sleep disorders as physical illnesses.

1951
Researchers at the University of Chicago discover rapid eye movement (REM) sleep, a stage in which the eyes move rapidly under the closed eyelids and the brain is busy in dream.

1929
Romanian neurologist Constantin Von Economo determines that sleep is regulated by the area of the brain known as the hypothalamus.

1832
In her book *Illustrations of Political Economy*, English essayist Harriet Martineau first suggests counting sheep as a cure for insomnia.

1937
The cinema's first narcoleptic, Sleepy, is featured in the Walt Disney Studios animated film *Snow White and the Seven Dwarves*.

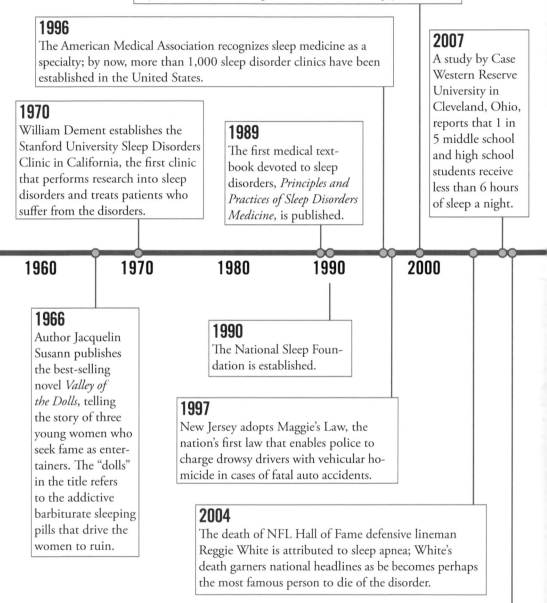

1999
By studying the DNA of dogs, researchers at Stanford University discover a common gene that causes narcolepsy in humans.

1996
The American Medical Association recognizes sleep medicine as a specialty; by now, more than 1,000 sleep disorder clinics have been established in the United States.

2007
A study by Case Western Reserve University in Cleveland, Ohio, reports that 1 in 5 middle school and high school students receive less than 6 hours of sleep a night.

1970
William Dement establishes the Stanford University Sleep Disorders Clinic in California, the first clinic that performs research into sleep disorders and treats patients who suffer from the disorders.

1989
The first medical textbook devoted to sleep disorders, *Principles and Practices of Sleep Disorders Medicine*, is published.

1960   1970   1980   1990   2000

1966
Author Jacquelin Susann publishes the best-selling novel *Valley of the Dolls*, telling the story of three young women who seek fame as entertainers. The "dolls" in the title refers to the addictive barbiturate sleeping pills that drive the women to ruin.

1990
The National Sleep Foundation is established.

1997
New Jersey adopts Maggie's Law, the nation's first law that enables police to charge drowsy drivers with vehicular homicide in cases of fatal auto accidents.

2004
The death of NFL Hall of Fame defensive lineman Reggie White is attributed to sleep apnea; White's death garners national headlines as be becomes perhaps the most famous person to die of the disorder.

2008
The National Sleep Foundation reports that 70 million Americans suffer from sleep disorders, including 60 million who are insomniacs.

Related Organizations

American Academy of Sleep Medicine

One Westbrook Corporate Center, Suite 920

Westchester, IL 60154

phone: (708) 492-0930

fax: (708) 492-0943

e-mail: inquiries@aasmnet.org

Web site: www.aasmnet.org

The American Academy of Sleep Medicine is the professional association of physicians who specialize in sleep medicine; the organization provides accreditation to physicians and sleep disorder clinics. Patients in need of sleep disorder treatment can follow a link on the academy's Web site to find physicians and clinics in their hometowns.

American Sleep Association

110 W. 9th St., Suite 826

Wilmington, DE 19801

fax: (940) 234-3357

Web site: www.sleepassociation.org

Founded by physicians, the American Sleep Association serves as a public information resource to educate patients and others about sleep disorders. By accessing the Sleep Encyclopedia on the organization's Web site, students can find explanations for each of the major sleep disorders as well as many more obscure and rare afflictions that interrupt people's sleep.

Association for Behavioral and Cognitive Therapies

305 7th Ave., 16th Floor

New York, NY 10001

phone: (212) 647-1890

fax: (212) 647-1865

Web site: www.aabt.org

The association represents therapists who provide cognitive behavioral therapy for people who suffer from many types of illnesses, including sleep disorders. Students who visit the association's Web site can find fact sheets on insomnia as well as bed-wetting, a parasomnia.

Brigham and Women's Hospital

Sleep Disorders Research

221 Longwood Ave., 036 BLI

Boston, MA 02115

fax: (617) 278-0863

Web site: www.brighamandwomens.org/sleepdisorders

Brigham and Women's Hospital is one of the nation's leading research institutions that concentrates on sleep disorders. Visitors to the hospital's Web site can find explanations for insomnia, sleep apnea, and other disorders; by accessing the link to "Sleep Smart: Finding Solutions to Common Disorders," students can learn about some of the polysomnograms employed to detect sleep disorders.

Centers for Disease Control and Prevention

Office of Communication

Building 16, D-42

1600 Clifton Rd. NE

Atlanta, GA 30333

phone: (800) 311-3435

e-mail: cdcinfo@cdc.gov

Web site: www.cdc.gov

The federal government's chief public health agency explores trends in diseases and other conditions that affect the health of Americans. By visiting the agency's Web site, students can find extensive information on many sleep disorders, including insomnia, narcolepsy, restless legs syndrome, and sleep apnea.

Harvard University Medical School Division of Sleep Medicine

401 Park Dr., 2nd Floor East

Boston, MA 02215

phone: (617) 998-8821

fax: (617) 998-8823

e-mail: sleep_medicine@hms.harvard.edu

Web site: http://sleep.med.harvard.edu

Harvard's Division of Sleep Medicine trains physicians in the latest therapies that address sleep disorders and provides seminars and similar events on treatment of sleep disorders for medical providers as well as members of the public. By visiting the Web site http://healthysleep.med.harvard.edu, students can find many resources on the science of sleep, such as how jet leg, caffeine, and aging affect sleep, as well as techniques on how to recognize sleep disorders and fight off insomnia.

National Center on Sleep Disorders Research

National Institutes of Health

Building 31, Room 5A48

31 Center Dr. MSC 2486

Bethesda, MD 20892

phone: (301) 592-8573

fax: (240) 629-3246

e-mail: nhlbiinfo@nhlbi.nih.gov

Web site: www.nhlbi.nih.gov/about/ncsdr/index.htm

The National Center on Sleep Disorders Research is the federal agency that provides funding for scientific research into sleep disorders. Visitors to the agency's Web site can take an interactive quiz testing their knowledge of sleep and sleep disorders and download research reports about sleep disorders.

National Highway Traffic Safety Administration

1200 New Jersey Ave. SE

West Building

Washington, DC 20590

phone: (888) 327-4236

Web site: www.nhtsa.dot.gov

The National Highway Traffic Safety Administration studies safety issues that relate to American highways. Visitors to the agency's Web site can access the National Survey of Distracted and Drowsy Driving Attitudes, which determined that a significant number of Americans lose their concentration and cause accidents because they drive while they are drowsy.

National Sleep Foundation

1522 K St. NW, Suite 500

Washington, DC 20005

phone: (202) 347-3471

fax: (202) 347-3472

e-mail: nsf@sleepfoundation.org

Web site: www.sleepfoundation.org

The National Sleep Foundation is the nation's leading educational and advocacy group for research into sleep disorders and treatment of the nation's 70 million citizens who suffer from insomnia and other disorders. Each year, the organization sponsors the annual Sleep in America poll, in which Americans are quizzed on their sleep habits and disorders. Results from the polls can be accessed at the organization's Web site.

Stanford University Hospital Sleep Disorders Clinic

Room 3301

Psychiatry Building

401 Quarry Rd.

Stanford, CA 94305

phone: (650) 723-6601

fax: (650) 725-8910

Web site: www.stanfordhospital.com/clinicsmedServices/clinics/sleep/sleep disorders

Founded in 1970 by William Dement, the Stanford University Hospital Sleep Disorders Clinic was the first clinic established specifically to study sleep disorders and provide treatment to patients. Visitors to the clinic's Web site can find facts and statistics about sleep disorders, while perspective patients can learn about the therapies they can expect to receive at the clinic.

For Further Research

Books

William C. Dement and Christopher Vaughan, *The Promise of Sleep: A Pioneer in Sleep Medicine Explores the Vital Connection Between Health, Happiness, and a Good Night's Sleep.* New York: Dell, 2000.

Gayle Greene, *Insomniac.* Berkeley and Los Angeles: University of California Press, 2008.

T. Scott Johnson, William A. Broughton, and Jerry Halberstadt, *Sleep Apnea: The Phantom of the Night.* Peabody, MA: New Technology, 2003.

Teofilo L. Lee-Chiong, ed., *Sleep: A Comprehensive Handbook.* Hoboken, NJ: Wiley-Liss, 2005.

Paul Martin, *Counting Sheep: The Science and Pleasures of Sleep and Dreams.* New York: Macmillan, 2005.

Michael L. Perlis, Carla Jungquist, Michael T. Smith, and Donn Posner, *Cognitive Behavioral Treatment of Insomnia: A Session-by-Session Guide.* New York: Oxford University Press USA, 2008.

Carlos Schenk, *Coping with Parasomnias: Overcoming Sleep Terrors, Sleep Paralysis, Sleep Eating, Sleep Walking, Sleep Sex, and Other Sleep Disorders.* Oakland, CA: New Harbinger, 2007.

Eluned Summers-Bremner, *Insomnia: A Cultural History.* London: Reaktion, 2008.

Bennett Alan Weinberg and Bonnie K. Bealer, *The World of Caffeine.* New York: Routledge, 2002.

Robert H. Yoakum, *Restless Legs Syndrome: Relief and Hope for Sleepless Victims of a Hidden Epidemic.* New York: Fireside, 2006.

Periodicals

Shazia Ahmad, "Generation Zzzzzz," *New York Observer*, April 25, 2005.

Clifton Brown, "Ex-Players Dealing with Not-So-Glamorous Health Issues," *New York Times*, February 1, 2007.

Cathleen F. Crowley, "Sleep Deprived: A Tired Fisherman Learns His Exhaustion Is Tied to Disorders," *Albany Times Union*, September 25, 2007.

Lawrence Epstein and Steven Mardon, "Homeroom Zombies," *Newsweek*, September 17, 2007.

William L. Hamilton, "Can't Sleep? Read This," *New York Times*, April 2, 2006.

William Hathaway, "Sleep-Deprived Teens Get Lower Grades, Exercise Less; a New Study Shows That Only About 20 Percent of American Adolescents Are Getting the Recommended Nine Hours of Sleep a Night," *Hartford Courant*, March 28, 2006.

Barbara Kantrowitz, Anne Underwood, and Karen Springen, "The Quest for Rest," *Newsweek*, April 24, 2006.

Mark Kram, "He Knew It Was Coming," *Philadelphia Daily News*, June 21, 2005.

Craig Lambert, "Deep into Sleep: While Researchers Probe Sleep's Functions, Sleep Itself Is Becoming a Lost Art," *Harvard Magazine*, July/August 2005.

Lynn Masters-Zaleski, "Night Terror," *Pediatrics for Parents*, November 2007.

Kathy McCleary, "In Search of Sleep," *Health*, September 2006.

Jon Mooallem, "The Sleep-Industrial Complex," *New York Times Magazine*, November 18, 2007.

Mehmet C. Oz, "How to Sleep Better," *Esquire*, April 2008.

Patrick Perry, "To Sleep, Perchance to Dream," *Saturday Evening Post*, July/August 2007.

Ron Winslow, "Their Duty Done, the Drowsy Dogs Can Doze Off Again; Stanford Pack Helped Solve the Mystery of Narcolepsy," *Wall Street Journal*, March 15, 2007.

Internet Sources

CBS News, "Waking Up to Drowsy-Driving Danger," October 20, 2004. www.cbsnews.com/stories/2004/10/20.earlyshow/contributors/melindamurphy/main650271.shtml.

Frontline, PBS, "Inside the Teenage Brain: From ZZZZZ's to A's," January 31, 2002. www.pbs.org/wgbh/pages/frontline/shows/teenbrain/from.

Jennifer Murphy, "How to Beat Jet Lag," KREN, Reno, Nevada, August 28, 2008. www.kren.com/Global/story.asp?S=8902770.

Nova scienceNOW, PBS, "Sleep," July 2007. www.pbs.org/wgbh/nova/sciencenow/3410/01.html.

Sheryl Rich-Kern, "Napping at Work Becoming Part of Corporate Culture?" New Hampshire Public Radio, August 6, 2008. www.nhpr.org/node/16986.

Anne Wollenberg, "Hypersomnia: My Doctor Thought I Was on Drugs," *London Independent*, July 29, 2008. www.independent.co.uk/life style/health-and-wellbeing/features/hypersomnia-my-doctor-thought-i-was-on-drugs-879317.html.

Source Notes

Overview

1. Quoted in Barbara Kantrowitz, Anne Underwood, and Karen Springen, "The Quest for Rest," *Newsweek*, April 24, 2006, p. 50.
2. Quoted in Kathy McCleary, "In Search of Sleep," *Health*, September 2006, p. 148.
3. Quoted in Paul Martin, *Counting Sheep: The Science and Pleasures of Sleep and Dreams.* New York: Macmillan, 2005, p. 258.
4. Quoted in Patricia McAdams, "The Science of Sleep," *Lancaster Intelligencer Journal*, March 20, 2006, p. 1.
5. Gayle Greene, *Insomniac.* Berkeley and Los Angeles: University of California Press, 2008, p. 142.
6. Quoted in *Charlie Rose Show*, "The Anatomy of Sleep and Sleep Disorders," MSNBC, June 5, 2006.
7. National Sleep Foundation, *Sleep-Wake Cycle: Its Physiology and Impact on Health*, 2006, p. 1.
8. Quoted in Christine Gorman, Dan Cray, Simon Crittle, Helen Gibson, and Grant Rosenberg, "Why We Sleep," *Time*, December 20, 2004, p. 46.
9. Quoted in McCleary, "In Search of Sleep," p. 148.
10. Quoted in McCleary, "In Search of Sleep," p. 148.
11. Quoted in Mark Kram, "He Knew It Was Coming," *Philadelphia Daily News*, June 21, 2005, p. 70.
12. Quoted in Jon Mooallem, "The Sleep-Industrial Complex," *New York Times Magazine*, November 18, 2007, p. 58.
13. Quoted in Sheryl Rich-Kern, "Napping at Work Becoming Part of Corporate Culture?" New Hampshire Public Radio, August 6, 2008. www.nhpr.org.
14. Quoted in Gorman, Cray, Crittle, Gibson, and Rosenberg, "Why We Sleep," p. 46.

What Are Sleep Disorders?

15. Greene, *Insomniac*, p. 28.
16. Quoted in Cathleen F. Crowley, "Sleep Deprived: A Tired Fisherman Learns His Exhaustion Is Tied to Disorders," *Albany Times Union*, September 25, 2007, p. E-1.
17. Anne Wollenberg, "Hypersomnia: My Doctor Thought I Was on Drugs," *London Independent*, July 29, 2008. www.independent.co.uk.
18. Wollenberg, "Hypersomnia."
19. Quoted in Margaret Webb Pressler, "Maybe It's Not So Cute," *Washington Post*, April 25, 2006, p. HE-1.
20. Quoted in Clifton Brown, "Ex-Players Dealing with Not-So-Glamorous Health Issues," *New York Times*, February 1, 2007, p. D-1.
21. Quoted in Jennifer Murphy, "How to Beat Jet Lag," KREN, Reno, Nevada, August 28, 2008. www.kren.com.
22. Quoted in Willow Lawson, "Nocturnal Perdition," *Psychology Today*, August 2003, p. 11.
23. Quoted in Lynn Masters-Zaleski, "Night Terror," *Pediatrics for Parents*, November 2007, p. 7.
24. Quoted in Donovan Vincent and Randy Starkman, "Sleepwalk Almost Kills Tennis Star," *Toronto Star*, April 5, 2006, p. A-1.
25. Quoted in Vincent and Starkman, "Sleepwalk Almost Kills Tennis Star," p. A-1.

What Causes Sleep Disorders?

26. Quoted in Rhonda L. Rundle, "Motion Sickness: Restless Legs Syndrome

Has Long Been Misdiagnosed and Misunderstood; That's About to Change," *Wall Street Journal*, June 20, 2005, p. R-5.

27. Quoted in Rundle, "Motion Sickness," p. R-5.

28. Quoted in Rundle, "Motion Sickness," p. R-5.

29. Greene, *Insomniac*, p. 161.

30. Quoted in Bennett Alan Weinberg and Bonnie K. Bealer, *The World of Caffeine.* New York: Routledge, 2002, p. 121.

31. Quoted in Viv Bernstein, "Signs of a Recovery," *New York Times*, September 28, 2003, p. 8-1.

32. Quoted in Ron Winslow, "Their Duty Done, the Drowsy Dogs Can Doze Off Again; Stanford Pack Helped Solve the Mystery of Narcolepsy," *Wall Street Journal*, March 15, 2007, A-1.

How Do Sleep Disorders Affect People?

33. Quoted in Lawrence Epstein and Steven Mardon, "Homeroom Zombies," *Newsweek*, September 17, 2007, p. 64.

34. Quoted in William Hathaway, "Sleep-Deprived Teens Get Lower Grades, Exercise Less; a New Study Shows That Only About 20 Percent of American Adolescents Are Getting the Recommended Nine Hours of Sleep a Night," *Hartford Courant*, March 28, 2006, p. A-4.

35. Quoted in BBC, "Junk Sleep Damaging Teen Health," August 27, 2007. http://news.bbc.co.uk.

36. Quoted in Craig Lambert, "Deep into Sleep: While Researchers Probe Sleep's Functions, Sleep Itself Is Becoming a Lost Art," *Harvard Magazine*, July/August 2005, p. 26.

37. Quoted in Lambert, "Deep into Sleep," p. 26.

38. Quoted in *West Australian*, "Sleep Deprivation Triggering Depression, ADHD: Expert," October 6, 2008. www.thewest.com.au.

39. Quoted in *West Australian*, "Sleep Deprivation Triggering Depression, ADHD."

40. Quoted in *Sleep Review*, "Sleep Apnea Raises Pregnant Women's Risk of Diabetes and Hypertension," June 6, 2007. www.sleepreviewmag.com.

41. Quoted in American Academy of Sleep Medicine, "New Study in Journal *SLEEP* Finds That Treating Insomnia Is Far Less Costly than Ignoring It," March 1, 2007. www.aasmnet.org.

42. Quoted in Associated Press, "Freeman in 'Good Sprits' After Surgery," MSNBC.com, August 5, 2008. www.msnbc.msn.com.

43. Quoted in CBS News, "Waking Up to Drowsy-Driving Danger," October 20, 2004. www.cbsnews.com.

44. Quoted in CBS News, "Waking Up to Drowsy-Driving Danger."

Can People Overcome Sleep Disorders?

45. Mehmet C. Oz, "How to Sleep Better," *Esquire*, April 2008, p. 120.

46. Quoted in Jennifer Corbett Dooren, "Talking Yourself to Sleep; Behavioral Therapies Teach Insomniacs to Snooze Without Relying on Drugs," *Wall Street Journal*, March 29, 2005, p. D-1.

47. Greene, *Insomniac*, p. 292.

48. Andrew Sullivan, "Adventures in the Sleep Lab," *Time*, December 20, 2004, p. 55.

49. Peter J. Hauri, Michael H. Silber, and Bradley F. Boeve, "The Treatment of Parasomnias with Hypnosis: A 5-Year Follow-Up Study," *Journal of Clinic Sleep Medicine*, June 15, 2007, p. 372.

50. Quoted in Patrick Perry, "To Sleep, Perchance to Dream," *Saturday Evening Post*, July/August 2007, p. 37.

51. William L. Hamilton, "Can't Sleep? Read This," *New York Times*, April 2, 2006, p. 9-1.

52. Quoted in Kantrowitz, Underwood, and Springen, "The Quest for Rest," p. 50.

List of Illustrations

List of Illustrations

Index

About the Author

Hal Marcovitz, a writer based in Chalfont, Pennsylvania, has written more than 100 books for young adult readers. His other titles in the Compact Research series include *Phobias, Hepatitis, Bipolar Disorders,* and *Meningitis.*